Rec'd. 7/14/88

RM

D1312289

DELIVERING MENTAL HEALTHCARE: A GUIDE FOR HMOs

John T. Boaz, M.D.

Pluribus Press, Chicago

RA
790.5
B57
cp.1

Library of Congress Catalog Card Number:
87-62423

International Standard Book Number:
0-931028-96-5

Pluribus Press, Inc.
160 East Illinois Street
Chicago, Illinois 60611

92 91 90 89 88   5 4 3 2 1

Printed in the United States of America

To my children,
Elizabeth and John

Contents

List of Tables

PREFACE

The primary purpose of this book is to serve as a practical guide for those who must evaluate, organize, develop, or market a department of mental health in a health maintenance organization (HMO). Throughout, the empirical rather than the theoretical has been emphasized, although references for further reading are included where indicated. The book has been designed for use as a handbook or a text on "how to" accomplish a certain set of tasks in prepaid mental health. If this is the extent of its usefulness, then the effort of writing it will have been worthwhile. However, I hope that the discussions, examples, and suggestions that comprise the text will be viewed in a broader context. Health care delivery in the United States is at a critical point: The old incentive system of fee for service is rapidly being replaced by a new system that is quite the opposite of traditional private practice incentives for reimbursement. The growth of prepaid health care is probably the most significant event in the history of American medicine, representing not only a radical change in financing but also in the increased emphasis given primary as opposed to secondary and tertiary prevention. Like a chain reaction, these changes will bring about a reevaluation of our entire system of health education. New questions will be asked: Are we training our health professionals in the most effective patterns of practice? Are we choosing applicants for professional schools who have ethical values and career goals that are consistent with the new system?

Mental health care delivery as part of general health care delivery cannot, nor should it attempt to, escape these radical changes. As medicine goes, so goes mental health. Therefore, this book can also be looked upon as an initial attempt to outline the new parameters of practice and professional attitudes that will be required in the mental health care delivery system of tomorrow. If the book is viewed in this broader context, then its usefulness will extend to students who are training for careers in mental health and to mental health professionals who realize that practical knowledge of prepaid mental health care is essential for their future.

John T. Boaz, M.D.

Chapter 1
AN OVERVIEW

Even the most casual social observer is aware that a revolution is occurring in American health care delivery. Health maintenance organizations (HMOs), representing what is called the prepaid health care field, are growing at a rate of 25 percent per year. By the year 2000 it seems likely that they will be the mainstream form of medical and mental health service delivery in the United States.

Despite the mushrooming of this vital industry, HMO mental health is a subject that to date has received little attention apart from governmental committee reports, professional journals, and narrowly focused articles in the popular press. For several reasons, little technical information regarding prepaid mental health care is easily accessible:

1. It is a new, burgeoning phenomenon on the American medical scene with, understandably, most of the energy of those involved being put into "doing" and not writing.

2. Practitioners of traditional fee-for-service psychotherapy have had no incentive to write constructively about a form of service delivery that has already reduced their practices by an average of 23 percent.[1]

3. Some in the prepaid sector do not believe that mental health is an essential element in their industry (at best, they see it as a costly but necessary nuisance, and at worst as the illegitimate offspring of neurology and theology—hence the less said about it the better).

4. The most important determinate for this lack of information is the embarrassing fact that the theoretical models in which most mental health practitioners were trained are totally inappropriate in a prepaid setting. The new workable models are just now being developed in HMOs, and it will probably take another five years for most training institutions to recognize them and reorient their programs.

A FUNDAMENTAL CONCEPT

At this point, let us pause and examine a fundamental concept in the delivery of prepaid mental health services: reverse incentive, or, more bluntly put, bigger is not better. This is actually a *key* concept in understanding how any HMO service functions, but is particularly germane to mental health. In order to understand reverse incentive, one needs only to sort through the legalese of any HMO subscriber policy to locate the clause(s) dealing with premium dollars and responsibility. Here always will be found a statement to the effect that for so many dollars per month the HMO agrees to provide or arrange for all basic health services and those supplemental health services covered in the contract. Note that the agreement is to provide and arrange for, not merely pay for. This is an essential distinction between a prepaid health insurance and an indemnity health insurance contract.

Worded in this manner, the agreement places the HMO at risk; that is, the HMO risks bankruptcy if the need for medical service, which it must provide, is greater than budgeted for by setting the premium at so many dollars per month. In other words, there is a financial incentive not to encourage unnecessary office visits, laboratory tests, and hospitalization, since there are only so many dollars per month to provide these services. This is the core of reverse incentive. Here, bigger truly is not better.

The traditional indemnity health insurance contract places no similar risk on health care providers. Indemnity contracts simply state that the insurance company will pay the providers of medical service so many dollars for a given procedure covered in the contract. If the number of monthly procedures results in a cost greater than the monthly premium, then that is the insurance company's headache and not the medical provider's. It can easily be seen that the indemnity insurance plan contains a financial incentive for the medical practitioner to encourage unnecessary office visits, hospitalizations, and laboratory tests. In point of fact, this is exactly what has happened in American medicine: A system of reimbursement that rewarded overutilization was created. We are just now beginning to estimate the damage caused by this system and to institute corrective action.

Those who condemn HMOs often use reverse incentive as ammunition in an attempt to prove that the prepaid sector renders second-rate, shoddy medical care. Their buzzword is underutilization, and their argument runs as follows: HMOs experience maximum profit in proportion to the number of office visits and laboratory tests that are not provided; in other words, the less they do, the bigger their profit. HMOs are therefore alleged to attempt, by whatever means they can, to avoid rendering needed medical treatment—treatment that is essential to the well-being of their subscriber members. To evaluate this argument, let's remind ourselves that the *M* in *HMO* stands for maintenance; a health maintenance organization will go bankrupt very quickly if it does not succeed in maintaining the health of its members, for the simple reason that the HMO is contractually responsible to provide or arrange for all necessary hospitalization of its members. The cost of providing a brief office visit starts at about $12; the cost of providing a day in hospital starts at about $300. It makes absolutely no financial sense, therefore, for the HMO to avoid rendering whatever medical treatment is necessary to promote a healthy and nonhospitalized membership. In sum, the argument for deliberate underutilization by HMOs is fatuous, since to ignore a legitimate medical problem in the office is to court fiscal disaster in the hospital.

IMPLICATIONS FOR MENTAL HEALTH CARE

How does all this apply to mental health treatment? A better way of phrasing that perhaps would be,"How does it *not* apply?" In mental health work, not only has the traditional system of indemnity insurance reimbursement rewarded overutilization but the very theories upon which most schools of psychotherapy are based require overutilization in order to be logically consistent. On one level, the statement "Mrs. Jones, you have a badly damaged ego; you'll have to see me three times a week for at least two years" stands as an indictment of a system of reimbursement, but at another level it accurately reflects a theoretical set that predates any form of insurance coverage for the treatment of emotional problems.

This theoretical set, which could be called the fee-for-service mentality, at its worst actively fosters a deemphasis of any attempt by the patient to rationally analyze and effectively deal with the reality-based stressors that are causing unpleasant emotional symptoms. A patient's legitimate complaints are deflected by suggesting that the present unsatisfactory situation is reminiscent of unpleasant past events, and that these events should be examined at length.

With a few exceptions (which will be discussed in another section), this fee-for-service mentality has prevailed for the past 80 years in the training institutions that produced, and are still producing, our psychotherapists, and in the popular press, which reinforces unrealistic expectations in the general population. The result has been the creation of a mental health service delivery system in which overutilization has been encouraged by most therapists and has been expected by most patients.

By keeping this situation in mind, it is not difficult to imagine the problems encountered in developing a high-quality and cost-effective HMO department of mental health. Therapists whose training and orientation are suited to HMO work are hard to find; once found, they must spend a great deal of their time educating patients as to what constitutes effective mental health care. But the rewards are well worth the struggle: a department of mental health whose outcomes demonstrate a suicide rate of zero; negligible hospitalization; and patients who have learned to cope effectively with their problems—all this at one-tenth the cost generated in the fee-for-service sector with an equivalent number of cases.

I am aware that this book may be considered controversial. It will undoubtedly "step on the toes" of traditional fee-for-service psychotherapists and irritate not a few HMO mental health department heads. It may also disturb some HMO managerial personnel (executive directors and medical directors) who have not been formally trained in mental health work and are therefore hesitant to ask such pointed questions as, "Who should run the department?" "Exactly how should they run it?" "Does what the department is doing make sense?"

The last two inquiries are of particular importance as HMO managers typically ask themselves, "Have I the right to tell mental health professionals how to conduct the department?" The answer is yes. If an individual has ultimate managerial responsibility for the quality and cost of service delivery in a department of mental health, then there are certain basics that he or she has the responsibility—and therefore the right—to insist upon. This does not mean that the manager is practicing psychiatry, psychology, or psychiatric social work. It simply means that there are a number of reasonable, commonsense policies and procedures that should be incorporated into the operation of any HMO department of mental health. The bottom line, of course, is that high-quality service at reasonable cost is a joint responsibility of management and the director of mental health.

TWIN IMPERATIVES OF THE FUTURE

As HMOs increase in number and size over the next decade, the imperative for cost containment and the simultaneous maintenance or improvement of quality of service will become more and more harsh. Managerial personnel are frequently unaware of the fact that departments of mental health are *extremely fertile* ground for significant cost savings, and in many cases, an actual increase in the quality of service. This potential may be overlooked or avoided by HMO managers for several reasons:

1. Mental health work is viewed as almost totally nonquantifiable and therefore not open to the kind of administrative review and critique that takes place in other departments such as medicine and pediatrics.

2. Few managers are aware of national average HMO mental health inpatient utilization rates, staffing ratios/mixes, or standards for provider productivity. They often accept

whatever rates, ratios, mixes, and productivity their departments generate, and therefore make costly errors.

3. If the manager is aware of these average figures, then he often sets the same expectations for his own department. In doing so, he again makes costly errors because the national average HMO mental health inpatient utilization rates are far in excess of what they should be, and staff ratios, mixes, and productivity standards remain far from ideal.

4. Unfortunately, an aura of mystery still envelops the field of mental health. Consequently, legitimate administrative inquiry and criticism are often defeated by avoidance tactics such as, "What do you want—suicides?" or "If we did that, we'd have umpteen lawsuits!" or "With a policy like that you'd have a staff of burnouts in six months."

And so it goes. The potential for cost savings combined with an increase in quality of service delivery remains unfulfilled. The mental health department becomes the forgotten service, bypassed for administrative review because positive change appears impractical or impossible.

The following chapters will examine some approaches by which this potential *can* be realized.

Chapter 2
THE DEPARTMENT: GENERAL CHARACTERISTICS

B efore we consider the who's and exact how's of managing an HMO department of mental health, let us examine some basic principles.

Regardless of the administrative structure and treatment model developed for a mental health department, the system must possess five characteristics: availability of service, accessibility of service, capacity, therapeutic effectiveness, and cost effectiveness. Although these characteristics are related and overlap, let us first consider them separately and then attempt to integrate them.

AVAILABILITY OF SERVICE

Availability of service is often made into an unnecessarily complex issue, sometimes by a director of mental health who wants to create a multiprovinced kingdom, but more often by HMO members (or their advocates, employee benefit representatives or employee assistance program personnel), who do not understand what good mental health care is. Good care does not require that a plethora of psychotherapeutic techniques be available. "What? You don't have psychoanalysis, hypnotherapy, biofeedback, primal therapy (etc., etc.)? I want an outside referral!" Don't fall into this trap of someone else's unrealistic expectations; go back to Public Law 93-222. This law was written with an adequate understanding of mental health needs. It requires that ambulatory services be available for diagnostic evaluation, crisis intervention, and referral.

What basic services must be available to meet these requirements? It is necessary and sufficient to provide emergency and routine evaluations, psychodiagnostic testing, and individual, couple, family, child and adolescent, and group therapy. If applied correctly, these essential evaluative and therapeutic modalities have the capability of resolving any emotional problem that is resolvable.

ACCESSIBILITY OF SERVICE

Accessibility of service refers to a system's potential for rapid response. How quickly can a patient be evaluated by a mental health provider after a request for mental health service has been made? How long does it take to get an appointment? These questions are crucial. It does no good to have a multitude of competent therapists backed up by many therapeutic modalities if the HMO's members have to wait three to six weeks for an initial appointment in mental health. If ambulatory services are not readily accessible to members in crisis, then the inpatient alternative becomes quite real to them and costly to the HMO. Therefore, any barriers to easy, direct triage by a mental health provider should be eliminated.

This statement obviously flies in the face of the "gatekeeper" concept so often invoked when trying to control the number of referrals to subspecialists. A gatekeeper may be appropriate in certain services such as allergy, cardiology, and plastic surgery, but not in mental health. Many HMOs have these policy/procedure checks on easy, direct access to a mental health provider. Examples of these guards against inappropriate utilization include requirements that all referrals to mental health be made by a primary provider; that only the member seeking mental health services can request an appointment; that lengthy evaluative questionnaires be completed by the member prior to his or her first appointment; or that financial disincentives in the form of large copayments be met prior to any service delivery. If an HMO has one or more of these restrictions to easy access, then perhaps it is time that it reevaluate the actual effect of these so-called cost-containment devices.

The family practitioner, internist, and pediatrician primary providers are not mental health professionals and should not be placed in the position of screening members' requests for mental health service. The only exception to this is the situation in which an effective liaison consultation model of service delivery has been created; that is, the primary providers have been taught to recognize and evaluate the exact degree of urgency of requests for mental health service. This arrangement requires many hours of in-service training and a more than average desire on the part of primary providers to acquire the needed skills of mental health work. If they are candid, most primary providers will tell you that they are uncomfortable trying to evaluate emotionally disturbed patients; they should be listened to.

The requirement that only the member seeking mental health service can request an appointment originated as a mechanism to monitor motivation and to prevent coercion of a person into the mental health system by his or her significant others. In its genesis within the public and fee-for-service sectors, this requirement made sense, but it is gratuitous in the prepaid sector. The HMO provider has no incentive to treat members who are not motivated or to coerce members into the system. I encountered an instance of this gatekeeping technique carried to an illogical extreme while on a consultation assignment. The HMO's department of mental health had refused to make an initial appointment for a psychotic 12-year-old girl because the patient did not call to schedule the appointment herself. Luckily, her parents had the good sense to take her to an emergency room, where authorization to hospitalize was ultimately received.

Gatekeeping, whether by means of evaluative questionnaires or by any other type of pretriage paperwork above and beyond minimum requirements to get a member to a mental health provider, is counterproductive. These questionnaires, used as screening devices, are intended to give diagnostic information and assist in determining how urgent a particular case is. The problem is that their administration and interpretation are time consuming and are almost always done by clerical rather than clinical staff. So by the time the clinician receives a written report stating that Mr. X is in crisis, Mr. X often is already in the hospital.

Surprisingly, there is still considerable debate in HMOs as to how large copayments for ambulatory mental health visits should be. Again, large copayments for ambulatory visits may be appropriate for some services, but not for mental health. The debate lingers because the specter of the bottomless pit phenomenon sticks in the minds of HMO actuaries. (But there is no bottomless pit; it's a leftover nightmare from the indemnity era.) Even if the initial visit is inappropriate, the HMO provider has not only the means but the incentive to make sure a second appointment is not scheduled. If a member in crisis is discouraged from making a mental health appointment by a 50 percent copayment, then he or she will go back home and attempt to cope, but a significant number of these members will decompensate and require hospitalization. Where is the cost savings then? It is more cost effective to generate 49 initial ambulatory visits that turn out to be inappropriate or unnecessary if the fiftieth is one in which a hospitalization can be avoided by early and energetic intervention.

What should HMO access times be? For the true psychiatric emergency in which a risk of suicide, homicide, or imminent decompensation requiring hospitalization exists, it should be possible for the member to be seen on the day of his or her request, ideally within an hour of presentation. For urgent but nonemergency cases, the waiting time should be no longer than 48 hours and for nonurgent, more routine problems, an appointment for evaluation should be available within 10 days.

The results of a recent national HMO mental health survey indicate that the prepaid sector is doing reasonably well in achieving short access times. Table 2-1 represents the overall average waiting times (with ranges) for emergencies, routine evaluations, and follow-up visits in group and staff model plans.

Table 2-1.
Overall Average and Range of Waiting Times for Service[2]

	Waiting Time	Range
Emergency	84.3% Same day	Same day to 7 days
Routine initial evaluation	13.7 days	2 days to 35 days
Follow-up visit	12.1 days	2 days to 32 days

Unfortunately, the survey did not report the average waiting times for urgent cases, but it did comment on the relationship between waiting times and a plan's mental health inpatient utilization: "... a relationship between access and hospital bed days was demonstrated for both routine initial evaluations and follow-up visits. Again, the results were predictable: Longer access times are associated with higher inpatient utilization."[2]

Question: What system of medical service delivery has the most rapid response rate (shortest access time)? Answer: emergency departments. In the crisis-oriented setting of an emergency department, the shaving of a few seconds from access time can, and often does, literally save lives. Here a multitude of triage techniques exist, all of them designed to eliminate any delay between the entry of a patient into the system and the medical evaluative process. Fortunately, only on rare occasions is the mental health department required to respond in so rapid a manner. Nevertheless, many emergency department triage procedures can be successfully adapted to HMO mental health work. For example, in very large departments a specific individual can be assigned to do emergency evaluations by telephone and in person; a technique a smaller department can use is the careful staggering of administrative time for its therapists in order to assure that a trained mental health therapist will be available during clinic hours to handle emergencies. (The issue of adapting techniques from other delivery systems will be covered in detail in the following chapter.)

DEPARTMENTAL CAPACITY

The issue of departmental capacity is a technically complex one involving not only staffing ratios but staff mix, provider productivity, and many other headache items for the director of the department and managerial personnel. These problems will be dealt with in detail in later sections; at this point, it is sufficient to state only that capacity relates to how long it takes to get a follow-up appointment after the initial mental health evaluation is complete. Having accessible service is useless if the department doesn't have the capacity for the ongoing treatment of the HMO's members, even in large numbers. A director who ignores the issue of departmental capacity may well be setting a course that will lead to under-utilization, a high hospitalization rate, and ultimate financial disaster.

How long should it take to get a follow-up appointment after the initial evaluation? Using the same criteria of urgency as we did with accessibility, the following holds true: It should be possible for emergency patients to be seen for at least a short follow-up appointment the next day. Urgent situations should have to be on hold no longer than one week, and routine problems should receive attention within two weeks.

THERAPEUTIC EFFECTIVENESS

Therapeutic effectiveness, the fourth required characteristic of a system for HMO mental health service delivery, is a thorny issue because there is no consensus in the mental health field as to what constitutes therapeutic effectiveness. Insight? Symptom reduction? Tranquil thoughts? Behavioral change? Reestablishment of chemical balance? A great deal of time can be wasted debating the pros and cons of the various criteria of therapeutic effectiveness. It is more practical to ask the question in a different way: Are there *common sense* criteria of therapeutic effectiveness? Obviously yes—that the deleterious effects of the emotional disturbance being treated be as brief and as slight as possible for both the patient and for those who are in association with him or her and that the disturbance not recur. Effectiveness therefore requires that the treatment system be timely, brief, educational, and comprehensive enough to include the patient's family, friends, and associates.

Let us consider each of these elements of therapeutic effectiveness in some detail.

Timeliness of intervention is clearly related to but

not synonomous with the previous topic of a system's rapidity of response (access time). Access centers on a department's ability to reduce waiting time to a minimum, whereas timeliness incorporates the added dimension of the patient's motivation. In a significant number of cases, patients request and receive a mental health evaluation but demonstrate insufficient motivation *at that time* to commit themselves to the work that successful therapy requires. It is fruitless to pursue such cases. If, on the other hand, the patient does have sufficient motivation for serious involvement, then that is the appropriate time for therapy to begin. Hesitancy by the therapist at this point is counterproductive: The patient is ready, and intervention is timely.

Brevity is not only the soul of wit, it also inhibits chronicity. Any school of therapy that advocates long-term therapy as the ideal is based upon the pessimistic assumption that those in need of mental health services are in some way flawed at the very core. This message is inevitably conveyed to the patients, making them feel even worse about themselves. Instead of encouraging patients to muster whatever personal resources they have remaining in a spirit of optimism and at least partial self-reliance, the proponents of long-term psychotherapy subtly (and often not so subtly) foster dependency and self-doubt and therefore potential chronicity and psychoinvalidism. Conversely, any theory that generates a short-term model of therapy as the ideal must, if it is to be ethical and logically consistent, assume that the patient is fundamentally intact. This is by far the best promise upon which to begin a case, even a case in which the patient's life seems to be in shambles. Both pessimism and optimism are contagious, so the initial inoculation should at least boost patients up a step rather than drag them down.

In considering the issue of comprehensiveness, we again encounter opposing views. Those who practice using a long-term model of psychotherapy will almost invariably insist that the so-called "identified patient" is the only legitimate focus of therapeutic endeavor. This view operationally translates into traditional individual long-term treatment. But here again, this fee-for-service stance ignores some commonsense observations that are backed up by a wealth of sociopsychological research: We are social animals, and we become symptomatic within the framework of our social units. We do not become emotionally distressed in a social vacuum that has no connection to the other individuals and groups who share our homes, workplaces, schools, etc. Therefore, therapeutic interventions should occur in the majority of cases at the level of the dysfunctional social unit and not at the level of some imaginary intrapsychic process.

This view opens up productive avenues of inquiry— just *who is* the patient? Perhaps the case of Mrs. Jones with the badly damaged ego could be reformulated with better results as a case requiring 10 joint sessions of marital counseling. It will certainly not benefit Mrs. Jones to be in individual therapy three times a week for two years if the primary stressor she faces is marital disharmony.

The requirement of effective psychotherapy that the emotional disturbance, once treated, not recur is, of course, an ideal, but ideals are worth persistent effort. Before this ideal is achieved, however, tremendous changes will have to occur not only in the dominant form of psychotherapy practiced in the United States but also in the prevalent attitudes of society at large regarding emotional distress and personal responsibility. This will require that psychotherapists be taught that their *ultimate* goal is the elimination of the need for their own services and that the general public be taught the principles of primary, secondary, and tertiary prevention. A long road at best. We must start somewhere, though, so let's go back to our HMO's model of service delivery. The model must structurally incorporate techniques for teaching the patient, the couples, and the families to rationally analyze how their distress came about, how it can be eliminated, and how similar disruptive situations can be avoided in the future.

COST-EFFECTIVENESS

A monograph published by the Federation of American Health Systems summarizes current data on mental health cost benefit research.[3] It substantiates what advocates of comprehensive mental health service in HMOs have sensed for some time:

■ Major studies of substance abuse programs uniformly show a benefit-to-cost ratio greater than one.

■ In experimental studies, patients receiving psychotherapy show a significant reduction in the use of other medical services.

■ According to an analysis of Blue Cross/Blue Shield claims files, total charges increased at a slower rate for beneficiaries receiving outpatient psychotherapy than for a comparable group with no outpatient visits. Furthermore, inpatient medical/surgical charges for persons 55 and over with at least seven outpatient psychotherapy visits were actually less than charges for the comparison group.

■ In hospital settings, surgical or medical patients provided with modest psychologically informed support had shorter stays and recovered more comfortably from surgery than those who did not receive such care.

These findings, the federal regulations regarding mental health services in qualified HMOs, and the trend toward more extensive state-mandated benefits all point to the inevitable conclusion that prepaid mental health is worthy of the concentrated efforts of the most creative managerial and clinical talent rather than being relegated to the status of second-class service and then forgotten. Once this conclusion is recognized and the talent assembled, what are the issues to be addressed in order to achieve cost-effectiveness? The primary issues are model of service delivery (which includes utilization review and control), type and size of provider staff, and benefits and exclusions. Unless these issues are addressed and resolved, there will be no "significant reduction in the use of other medical services" and no "benefit-to-cost ratio greater than one."

Chapter 3
MODEL OF SERVICE DELIVERY

As indicated in chapter 1, the traditional models in which most mental health practitioners were trained are totally inappropriate in a prepaid setting. The fee-for-service mindset of these practitioners produces conflict in those required to do brief therapy, crisis intervention, and a great deal of group work while maintaining a low hospitalization rate, easy accessibility, and high member satisfaction. Add to this the overt and covert criticism they receive from their colleagues in private practice and the stress of working with a mandated population in the face of specific limitations in coverage and you have fertile ground for such problems as therapist burnout, low provider productivity, high staff turnover, and poor interdepartmental relations.

During the past decade, mental health care providers in HMO settings have forged some new models of service delivery that may well be the norms for the field of mental health in this country by the year 2000. These new models generate low hospitalization rates, high member and employer satisfaction, negligible rates of suicide and malpractice suits, and cost-effective operational patterns. As in any innovative endeavor, there is disagreement on points of theory, procedure, and emphasis among the innovators, but the following elements are representative of their views:

1. Emphasis is placed on available, easily accessible ambulatory service as opposed to inpatient care.

2. Emphasis is placed on short-term specific goal-oriented therapy as opposed to traditional long-term insight-oriented therapy.

3. Crisis intervention services are emphasized.

4. Therapy is oriented toward the dysfunctional social unit concept rather than the traditional "identified patient" concept.

5. The role of group therapy as a cost- and therapeutically effective modality is fully recognized.

6. Smoothly functioning interfaces between mental health and other departments within the HMO, both medical and administrative, are considered to be of vital importance.

7. Thorough knowledge of and full utilization of available community resources are stressed.

8. The traditional "50-minute hour" is not necessarily accepted as the standard work unit in HMO mental health.

9. In keeping with the principle of primary prevention, a psychoeducative approach to service delivery is emphasized.

10. A documented quality assurance program that addresses structure, process, and outcome must be developed and implemented.

11. The difficult task of developing comprehensive but easily implementable written departmental policies and procedures must be performed.

12. Mechanisms for accurate utilization review and effective utilization control must be developed and implemented.

13. The mental health staff provides care that is *needed*, not care that is faddish or simply wanted.

14. The concepts of consumer responsibility and patient compliance are emphasized throughout the system.

15. In recognizing the unique stresses associated with mental health work, a system of mutual staff support in the form of staff meetings and case consultations must be provided.

16. In staff selection, the important concepts of role

equivalency and "HMO compatibility" are recognized.

17. The concept of continuity of care is emphasized.

ENTERING THE SYSTEM

Using these 17 items as basic building blocks of an HMO model of service delivery, let us examine a functioning department by assuming the role of a *very* emotionally disturbed member at the point of entering the system. One of the more productive techniques in good therapy is to at least occasionally ask oneself, "How would I feel if I were the patient?"

Imagine that you are in good physical health but have slept only four hours of the previous 48 hours. You're exhausted, you anxiety is sky-high, and you are developing a tremor in both hands. It's 11 a.m. You are at work, but it's impossible to concentrate or make even the simplest of decisions. The thought "I'm going crazy" starts intruding repeatedly into your consciousness as objects and individuals in the office begin to look more and more strange. A tight situation.

Then you think, "Hey, I've got mental health coverage with that HMO I just signed up for! I've got to do something, and now!" You call the HMO. This is the point at which the prepaid wheat is winnowed from the prepaid chaff: If you're told anything other than some equivalent of, "Knock off work and come by the department; you'll be seen today," then you've got real troubles. For example, "This is a recording; there is no one available at present to. . ." or "Yes, I understand your sense of urgency, but our first opening isn't until..." or "Oh, you'll be seen today all right; you'll come in and take some tests, and then we'll schedule you to see Dr. Krankenhaus...let's see... yes, next Tuesday at 10 a.m." What would you do at this point? There is a slim possibility you could get in through your HMO's emergency walk-in clinic, but chances are they will only refer you to the mental health department, where you'll probably encounter, "This is a recording..." or some such.

Your choices are now the fee-for-service sector (either a private practitioner or an emergency department), a community mental health center, or toughing it out. The last choice might, but probably won't, prevent decompensation and therefore hospitalization or worse. You might, but probably won't, be seen on such short notice by a private practitioner, but even if you were, he or she would probably recommend hospitalization, which would have to be authorized by the HMO, and since it's only 12:15 p.m., the utilization control person (assuming contact can be made) probably will require that you call the HMO's mental health department for an evaluation. You can probably be seen in the local community clinic, but chances are no psychiatrist will be available, and because you're more than likely going to require a short course of medication, the clinic probably will either send you home with verbal support or recommend hospitalization—which again brings up the problem of authorization and sends you back to the starting line. You can certainly be seen in an emergency room by a physician, but it may take from one to six hours because the triage hierarchy ranks gunshot wounds and pulmonary emboli higher than impending psychosis. The physician then will either sedate you and send you home or put you in a holding unit and recommend hospitalization. The first course of action will leave you facing a repeat performance in the system on the following day; the second course will likely land you in the hospital. It may not be an approved hospital, so you'll have to be transferred in a day or two after you've been "stabilized," but ah . . . at last you're safe!

This is only a partial scenario of the horrors associated with a phenomenon known as "falling through the cracks" of the mental health system. It's expensive, not therapeutic, and, unfortunately, not that uncommon, even in the prepaid sector. However, in a properly conducted HMO department of mental health, things like this do not occur because easily accessible ambulatory service and crisis intervention are emphasized.

What does "are emphasized" mean operationally? It means that someone, preferably a mental health provider, would have been available to take the above call, evaluate the degree of urgency, and in this case, schedule an evaluation with physician backup for medication (not necessarily a psychiatrist) within three hours.

As mentioned in chapter 2, large departments (those serving over 100,000 members) can accomplish this by hiring as a triage officer a mid-level provider such as a psychiatric social worker with good medical evaluative skills or a bachelor's level nurse with extensive mental health experience. His or her primary tasks would be to screen incoming requests for service by telephone or in person and make the required disposition. Some requests will be inappropriate for the mental health department; therefore, this person must have full working knowledge of the medical and administrative resources of the HMO and the community for purposes of referral. Because other possible dispositions include immediate inpatient or partial hospitalization, procedures for authorization and transport must be in place and functioning smoothly. Some encounters will require medication, so the triage officer must have easy access to a physician. In some cases, a follow-up appointment the next day will be necessary. It is here that no popularity prizes will be awarded by other staff members: If an appointment is not available, it must be created. For example, a provider is told that a 3 p.m. slot the next day that just opened by cancellation is now filled with an emergency follow-up, that a 20-minute block between the 10 a.m. and 11 a.m. sessions the next day must be opened for a quick follow-up, or even that 30 minutes of administrative time for the next day is now clinical time. Another important but stressful element of triaging is evaluating and disposing incoming requests from emergency departments, private practitioners, employee assistance program representatives, school administrators, and others for hospitalization of members. Triaging is often a rescue and retrieval operation involving tedious explanations of benefit restrictions, exclusions, and member compliance standards. It is surprising how many "actively suicidal" members undergo immediate spontaneous remissions and are able to come in for an evaluation when the private practitioner learns that there is a chance hospitalization would not be covered.

The triage officer should not be burdened with the job of departmental scheduling, because that would be confusing clerical with clinical tasks. He or she should, however, be given additional assignments that can be interrupted easily—for example, the collection and collation of utilization review data and chart review for quality assurance meetings. Framed in this manner, the job of triage officer can be one of the most cost-effective positions in the department. A note of caution: The stress associated with this position can lead to rapid burnout if the person is not chosen wisely or is not given a clear job description. Prior successful emergency department experience is a double plus on a resumé here. A way to avoid potential burnout is to rotate the position among three or four mid-level providers over the span of a week or two. Even though there may be lowered expertise and occasional confusion about "who's on call," these problems are more easily dealt with than burnout.

On the other end of the scale, in small HMOs of 20,000 to 30,000 members, it probably will not be cost effective to assign one full-time employee (or equivalent) to triaging. An exception to this would be an HMO with a membership consisting primarily of members with very low socioeconomic status or on Medicaid. Here, a typical pattern of utilization is the eleventh-hour crisis presentation, which can require a full-time equivalent triage position in order to avoid a *very* high hospitalization rate. In these smaller demand situations, adequate coverage can be achieved by scheduling provider administrative time with no overlapping; that is, administrative time is carefully staggered so that one provider is at least nominally free at all times to do triage work.

Whether the department is large or small, a great deal of triaging actually is done by mental health secretaries, either alone or with the assistance of whatever provider is available at the time. From a legal point of view, this is a risky situation, and there are no clear-cut guidelines to follow. A rule forbidding clinical decisions by clerical staff seems reasonable, but the decision not to interrupt a provider who is triaging on the telephone when another emergency call comes in *is* a clinical decision. Who knows what the second caller will do while waiting to be contacted? In court, any contact the secretary had with a patient can be construed to have had a detrimental effect.

There is no way around it: The mental health secretary is a key person on the treatment "team." As such, this person's selection should never be left to chance, to a well-meaning personnel representative, or to anyone who is not well versed in mental health service delivery needs. Above and beyond the usual secretarial skills, mental health secretaries must be able to:

- Relate with ease to highly disturbed or confused members who present in crisis either on the telephone or in the clinic

- Recognize the "true emergency" on the telephone or in person (even if the member presents with a facade of nonchalance) and make sure that the member comes to the attention of a provider *immediately*

- Respond with great sensitivity to the unique and confidential nature of mental health work; all medical service is confidential, but mental health work abounds in unusual pitfalls in the area of confidentiality.

Even if the secretaries have had prior experience in mental health, they should be required to meet performance standards incorporating the skills noted above and should be given in-service training.

In summary, gaining entry to the system can be a

disruptive process itself unless providers are available as needed. Considerable damage can occur to both the member and the HMO's budget if "cracks" are allowed to develop at the entry point of the system.

STEP 2 INTO THE SYSTEM

Assuming that the very disturbed member mentioned earlier got a same-day appointment with no unnecessary paper work, what happened then? Once the member is in the system, a variety of things can happen, some beneficial and others not. The thing to keep in mind at this point is that once the member has entered the system, the full range of departmental services can be brought to bear in a selectively therapeutic manner. Outcome will depend mainly upon three variables: the orientation and efficiency of the department, the competence and morale of the therapist, and the resources (both internal and external) and motivation of the member.

In order to examine the process of treatment modality selection and outcome, I would like to describe two presentations that I have experienced. Both have been sufficiently altered to protect confidentiality without obscuring the essential principles of prepaid mental health service delivery that they demonstrate. The first case is the example presented earlier.

Case 1

Upon examination, the member was found to be a 24-year-old single male who had recently received an M.B.A. degree and moved across the country to start his present job six weeks prior to this "episode." Although he had attempted to make friends at work, the company was small, and most of the other employees in his office were middle-aged, married, and felt that they had little in common with him. He had thought about a dating service or joining a singles' organization, but he was, as he described himself, shy. As a result, his life settled into the routine of office and apartment, with marked social isolation, loneliness, low self-esteem, and now the symptoms of insomnia, extreme anxiety, derealization, and a sense of despair. His past history was helpful in that it revealed that he had been able to make a few friends in college, had never abused alcohol or used drugs, enjoyed camping, and had never experienced similar symptoms. What's to be done with him? Major tranquilizers? Hospitalization? Or something else?

The therapist contacted a psychiatrist in the department who reviewed the case findings and saw the member for a short medication evaluation. A small amount of sedative medication (enough for one night) was prescribed and a follow-up appointment was scheduled for the next day.

At follow-up, the member was much more calm, having slept more than 15 hours. This second session was used for further evaluation and working out a treatment plan with the member. Both therapist and member agreed that the primary stressors precipitating the symptoms were loss of family and other social support due to moving, the pressure of a first job, and the present intense social isolation and loneliness. The member claimed that he had always had some difficulty in making friends, describing himself as "socially inept." Various activity groups where he could meet others and make friends were discussed; because of his interest in camping, the member chose to investigate joining the American Youth Hostel Association. To provide a matrix of emotional support and training in developing social skills in this period of transition, the therapist suggested that the member also begin attending a mixed therapy group held weekly at the clinic. Here some resistance was encountered: He would be fearful of talking in a group; group therapy wasn't as good as individual therapy. But after an explanation of exactly how the group was conducted and why the experience might be very beneficial, he agreed to try it.

Results? As predicted, the group therapy sessions provided the young man not only some much-needed human contact but also a nonthreatening environment in which he was successful in reducing his "shyness" and "social ineptness." At the same time, he enrolled in sailing classes offered by the youth hostel group and became active in their outings, making some friends in the process. In fact, he became so active that he informed the therapy group after three months that he was going to "try it on my own." This decision was supported, and in the final group session he articulated his own formula to prevent recurrence of a similar episode: Good friends are good medicine.

Discussion. This case demonstrates several characteristics of prepaid mental health service delivery that are of benefit to members and the HMO.

The rapidity with which the member gained access to a system with good capacity for follow-up not only prevented any further deterioration in his condition but likely averted a hospitalization as well. Most fee-for-service providers would have recommended hospitalization for a patient who demonstrated severe anxiety, agitation, and derealization. In this case, the emphasis on easy access, crisis intervention techniques, and the capacity for quick follow-up paid off for both the member and the HMO.

It should also be noted that the therapist worked directly with the member to develop a treatment plan, that the plan addressed actual here-and-now stressors in the member's life, and that the treatment plan had a psychosocial base. Working directly with the member made sense because the member was actually a partner in the transaction.

This case also demonstrates the value of using available community resources, of thinking collaboratively: What individuals or organizations can be of assistance? Here the youth hostel organization served to assist the member in integrating himself in a compatible social network, thereby reducing the stresses associated with loneliness and low self-esteem. Operationally, "thorough knowledge and full utilization of available community resources" (point 7 in the service delivery model above) means that each provider has the equivalent of a community resource handbook, knows how to use it, and actually uses it. If such a handbook is not available, then the department should develop one. This is a time-consuming operation, but it will quickly pay for itself many times over. Simply compile listings (name, address, telephone number, services available, and contact person, if possible) of organizations or agencies in the HMO's service area that deal with the problems of child abuse, family violence, substance abuse, social isolation, etc., and make this information available to members when indicated. This information should always be accompanied by an explanation to the member of exactly how the resource referral will be of benefit. The axiom that "good mental health work is in great measure good social work" is nowhere more clearly demonstrated than in the HMO's comprehensive use of community resources.

Finally, one of the most important treatment modalities in prepaid mental health care is demonstrated in this case by the use of group therapy to provide the member emotional support and education in developing needed social skills. Every HMO should have an active group therapy program. There are no "carved in stone" rules that apply here, but up to (and even beyond) 40 percent of total mental health encounters can occur in group settings with high member acceptance, low risk, good outcome, and significant savings. The initial objections by the member in this case—that he would be afraid to talk in a group, and that group therapy isn't as good as individual therapy—are typical and must be addressed. Care must be taken to explain to the member that group therapy not only is an effective treatment modality but is often the treatment of choice. Group therapy provides a nonthreatening educational opportunity that reflects reality to a much greater extent than does traditional one-on-one therapy. Again, we are social animals, and we become emotionally distressed in the contexts of our social units. What better way to correct this distress than in the therapeutic social context of group therapy?

Group therapy is also an extremely cost-effective

treatment modality.[4] The potential reduction in provider clinical time brought about by an active and extensive group therapy program will average 55 percent or more compared to the time required to treat the same number of members individually. The average number of individual mental health encounters generated by an HMO member is six. Therefore, an average of six hours of provider time per referred member will be required if treatment is rendered via the traditional 50-minute hour. The average number of group therapy encounters generated by an HMO member is 15. Therefore, assuming an average of nine members per one and one-half-hour group, the amount of provider time required to deliver service to a member is two hours and thirty minutes, or 42 percent of six hours—a savings in provider clinical time of 58 percent.

The groups should be designed to address multiple needs of the membership; therefore, they should be of various types—open-ended heterogeneous, time-limited heterogeneous, and time-limited homogeneous groups for specific tasks (couples' groups, women's groups, parenting groups, etc.). These groups should range in size from 8 to 14 members and be conducted by one therapist (with the exception of training a provider to conduct a specific group, having a cotherapist is simply another method of "gilding the lily" and should be avoided).

The previously cited national HMO mental health survey also reported results on the current use of group therapy. Table 3-1 represents the average distribution of caseload by various treatment modalities (with ranges) for group and staff model plans.[2]

Table 3-1.
Average Distribution of Caseload by Treatment Modality[2]

	Percent of Caseload	Range
Individual	61.4	35–91
Group	5.5	0–30
Family	6.2	1–25
Couple	8.9	1–40
Medication checks	13.1	1–50
Other	4.9	1–10

In my opinion, the 5.5 percent of the caseload now being seen in group therapy could—and should—be increased to at least 25 to 30 percent. However, changes of this sort may be slow in appearing because resistance to group therapy is not unique to members; many providers still cling to the mistaken notion that *ipso facto*, individual therapy is best in all situations.

Case 2

This case presented as a nonemergency, routine request but demonstrates, among other things, some of the difficulties HMO providers encounter in the area of unrealistic expectations.

The member, a 37-year-old college-educated housewife with three children, after completing the departmental intake form, requested that the secretary give her an authorization for 20 visits to an "agoraphobia clinic" that was conducting a newspaper and television marketing campaign in the city at the time. The secretary informed her that she would have to discuss outside referrals with the therapist. This irritated the member. Her irritation was still evident when she came to the therapist's office for the initial evaluation. "I want an authorization for my 20 visits.... I've got agoraphobia and this clinic specializes in that," she said, producing a newspaper ad for the clinic. The therapist carefully explained the HMO's policy governing outside referrrals, but that wouldn't do. She demanded the authorization and finally left the office abruptly, threatening legal action.

That afternoon, the therapist received a call from the member's husband requesting clarification. In the course of the telephone conversation, it became clear that this was a multiproblem family attempting unsuccessfully to deal with child-rearing difficulties and marital disharmony. A conjoint appointment for the couple the following week was suggested by the therapist and accepted by the husband.

The first 25 minutes of the appointment the following week were spent in again explaining the plan's policy regarding outside referrals, acknowledging that problems certainly existed in the family, and encouraging the couple to take advantage of the services that were available to them. As the session progressed, the logic of the therapist's suggestions began to have an impact. The couple agreed to return the following week. After two more conjoint sessions and one family session attended by the children, the situation had become much clearer to both the therapist and the couple. Their marriage had deteriorated over the previous four to five years; the husband had withdrawn from involvement in the home, especially in matters of child rearing, leaving the wife to face the task of raising their children with increasing feelings of frustration, irritability, and, finally, panic episodes. The children, who were essentially normal but very intelligent and active, responded to the decrease in effective parental guidance by increased limit testing.

By this time, the couple had developed confidence in the therapist and were willing to assist in formulating a treatment plan that addressed both the marital and child-rearing difficulties. They agreed to attend a weekly, one and one-half-hour couples group scheduled to start at the clinic in three weeks. They also agreed to enroll in a 12-week series of classes in child rearing given at a local high school using the STEP (Systematic Training for Effective Parenting) program as a model.

Results? Both parents were, fortunately, well motivated and took full advantage of each program. They used the couples group to explore their own relationship and recapture a sense of communality, shared goals, and mutual affection. The child-rearing classes were also quite helpful to them. Here they not only learned valuable techniques in child rearing, but also the fact that really successful parenting is by definition best accomplished as a joint venture. This recognition, which they had lacked, brought them even closer together. They terminated treatment in a final conjoint session with a sense of achievement and praise for the therapist's conduct of their case.

Discussion. Here, as in the first case, we see the productive use of community resources and group therapy in bringing about a satisfactory resolution to a disruptive and potentially dangerous situation. We see something else, too. The wife's initial misunderstanding of the etiology and proper treatment of her condition, and her insistence on her "right" to be allowed to pursue an inappropriate course of treatment are indicative of two disturbing facts of which HMO mental health providers must be aware: The general public has several misconceptions as to the causes and effective treatment of emotional distress, and information regarding the rights and responsibilities of HMO members is, in many instances, not being communicated to new subscribers. The first is a problem in public health education. The second is a problem in HMO marketing and member education. Both problems, however, result in very distorted and unrealistic member expectations that the mental health provider must correct if high quality service is to be delivered.

One does not need to be a mental health professional to see that the woman's self-diagnosis and demand for an outside referral to an agoraphobia clinic were strategies to avoid confronting the primary area of conflict and stress—her marriage. It is a moot point whether this avoidance was "conscious" or "unconscious." Most individuals who present with disturbing symptoms *do* have at least a general notion of their cause. They choose to ignore or deemphasize this knowledge because they feel that the risk of open and direct confrontation is too great. (The wife in this case admitted in a session of the couples group that she had not sought marriage counseling initially because she feared the consequences of a divorce if marriage counseling failed.) This attitude is an example of opting for apparent short-term gains over the more difficult and hazardous commitment required for any satisfactory resolution of interpersonal conflict.

This form of "short-sightedness" is quite common in the general population. It has been accentuated in recent years by the mass media and many fee-for-service mental health professionals who encourage the views that symptoms arise without any connection to what is occurring in the person's life *at that time*, and that these isolated symptoms can be successfully treated by "specialists" without any reference to those current life stresses.

The trend toward superspecialization became evident several years ago when ads started appearing in the newspapers and on the radio announcing the opening of services devoted to the treatment of eating disorders, agoraphobia, panic disorders, psychogenic pain, kleptomania, grief, and other disturbances. Radio and television talk shows featured experts who alerted the general public to the prevalence and danger of these disorders. Popular magazines ran full-length articles by these experts recycling what had already been said on the air.

Although no statistics are available regarding how successful these marketing strategies were, the fact that they continue is an indication that they were not without some effect in maintaining or increasing "market share." However, two other results of these strategies should be examined. The first is their effect on the general public's perception of emotional distress and the second is their effect on mental health service delivery in HMOs. The effects are interrelated and both are mischievous.

No argument is set forth here against advertising (any supporter of HMOs would be on very thin ice objecting to advertising). The objection to *this sort* of advertising is that it fragments any rational theory of comprehensive service delivery and therefore misleads the public. It totally ignores the fact that a symptom cannot exist *in vacuo,* that it can only exist as one facet of a global distress syndrome that has been precipitated by real stresses coming from the real world. By shifting the focus away from a general field theory of emotional distress, the superspecialist's advertising leads the layman into compartmentalizing his or her self-image. In that direction lies chaos—chaos in terms of an increase in unproductive anxiety and an increase in unrealistic expectations of what effective, comprehensive mental health services can actually provide.

It is in this area of increased unrealistic expectations that the HMO mental health provider encounters difficulty. A great deal of extra time must be spent explaining to members, "Yes, you're 10 pounds overweight, and yes, you become anxious in public places, but no, you don't require a specialist in eating disorders and another in panic disorders for the proper treatment of your condition." Even when the explanation is apparently accepted, that isn't always the end of the story. The member will often reintroduce the issue of specialization and outside referral in the course of therapy as a resistance to continuing in treatment.

Fortunately, HMOs are in a better position to correct these effects than some may think. They can not only correct them, but at the same time can increase their enrollment and foster a good public image of HMOs in general. In order for this to happen, mental health directors must be willing to adapt two community mental health center (CMHC) techniques to HMO use, and executive and marketing directors must be willing to spend some extra money in nontraditional marketing campaigns.

CMHCs are mandated to provide both consultation/education and outreach services to agencies and individuals within their service areas. Prepaid mental health departments are ideal vehicles by which to synthesize and present the most useful elements of consultation/education and outreach activities. For example, the mental health staff can determine the principal problem issues in the HMO's service area by direct observation in the clinic and from information supplied by local agencies and organizations such as departments of social service, police departments, protective services, churches, etc. When the major problem issues have been identified (for example, alcoholism, child abuse, or chronic overspending), then a designated individual in the department can contact local churches, high schools, colleges, and business and social clubs. These organizations are usually happy to sponsor a talk on stress management, child rearing, or substance abuse. Also, newspapers and radio stations are often more than willing to give space or time to a well-presented mental health topic. Exposure of this sort has two beneficial effects: It provides the public with information about the causes and proper treatment of emotional distress and, at the same time, displays the prepaid sector in a very positive light.

Because the "payoff" is not immediate, only a few HMOs have been far-sighted enough to explore these techniques of combined public education and marketing. Plans that have done so apparently do not regret their adventurousness, since they continue to take the risk of providing this much-needed service.

Rights and responsibilities are inevitably linked, a fact that is not sufficiently stressed in most HMO mental health marketing and member education. From the point of view of marketing directors, this deficiency is understandable: They want limited mental health benefits that appear unlimited when marketed. This practice places the provider in an uncomfortable position and creates unnecessary hostility in the subscriber. It also wastes valuable clinical time, inasmuch as it is the provider who usually has to explain the "lock-in" clause of an HMO service contract to a disappointed and angry member. Case 2 demonstrates this dilemma quite well.

At least a partial solution to the problem of lack of clarity in coverage provisions may lie in a rethinking of marketing strategies in the light of a reevaluation of potential member acceptance. Although I certainly don't have hard data to back up the assertion, it is my impression, gained through nine years of work developing two HMO departments of mental health, providing direct service, and consultation work in HMO mental health, that simple but clear explanations of plan limitations and member responsibilities would be accepted by employer and union benefit representatives. If the product is good, it can be displayed with confidence. It is likely that marketing directors have more latitude than they may think to begin the task of member education as early as the initial selling stage.

Chapter 4
STAFFING

One of the most important maxims to remember when recruiting providers is that quality assurance and utilization control begin with staff selection. Before the issues of degrees, resumés, or references are considered, think of HMO compatibility—how well suited is this person to work in an HMO? Among various methods by which this question can be answered accurately, one of the best is the preemployment interview.

INTERVIEWING

First, applicants should be questioned on what they already know about prepaid mental health care. If the applicant is knowledgeable and comfortable with the concepts of reverse incentive, short-term therapy, crisis intervention, and the rational allotment of resources from having worked in an HMO or community mental health center or from reading about the prepaid sector, this is a very positive sign. Such applicants are rare, however, so the question becomes one of trainability.

Applicants should be given some hypothetical case presentations and asked to formulate treatment plans. Their responses should be carefully noted. Can they formulate the case in order to reach the stage of treatment planning? If not, the interview should be terminated. If they can conceptualize the case, is their treatment plan sprinkled with such words as "intensive individual," "long-term," "insight oriented," or "uncovering unconscious motivation," with no mention of alternative formulations even if they are prompted toward these alternatives? If so, these practitioners would not be comfortable in an HMO setting.

Another type of applicant to be wary of are the therapists who have recently given up failing private practices. They often make a good impression in an interview but usually can't stand up under close questioning regarding the specifics of their own practice— how they conducted family therapy, how they feel about brief versus long mental health leaves of absence from work. Invariably, the fee-for-service ethos will surface here if it is present. Again, these therapists would not be comfortable in an HMO.

Another informative technique in preemployment

interviewing is to ask prospective providers what theorists or writers in the field have influenced them the most. If they can't give even one name associated with a psychosocial or community-oriented approach to therapy, then they should be hired only with extreme hesitation.

A foolproof method of conducting preemployment evaluations for mental health workers is to sit in while they screen an incoming nonemergency case. (Note: You should check with your legal counsel before adopting this technique to make sure you are on firm ground.) The applicant simply is introduced by name and the member is told what is going to happen and asked if he or she has any objections. If there are no objections, the interviewer sits back and observes carefully. Does the applicant put the member at ease? Does he or she elicit enough information to formulate the case and draw up a treatment plan in a reasonably short time? Does the prospective provider terminate the interview at the appropriate point? After the member has left the office, the applicant is asked to recapitulate the essentials of the case and formulate a treatment plan. This is the acid test, an actual sample of performance. Obviously, such an interview can provoke anxiety in the applicant, and this should be taken into consideration. Nevertheless, the primary concern still must be whether this person's performance would be acceptable in this HMO's department of mental health. For fifteen years I have routinely conducted this form of preemployment evaluation in both HMOs and CMHCs and have noted that applicants who "passed" and were hired invariably did well, but that applicants who "failed" but were hired for other reasons did poorly.

An ancillary but useful technique in screening applicants for acceptability in the department is to conduct at least part of the interview with as many other staff members present as possible. This gives each of them the opportunity to ask questions and form an impression. Their impressions and observations should be heeded carefully; after all, they are the ones who would be working most closely with the prospective staff member. However, this process is not simply a democratic courtesy. The staff can often ferret out subtle deficiencies that might be missed in a one-on-one approach. Part of what they do for a living is detecting hidden agendas.

These approaches to interviewing applicants may seem rather harsh, even brutal, if one does not consider the consequences of bringing on someone who disagrees with and will resist learning the basic tenets of HMO mental health work (see chapter 3). If they don't have these necessary concepts of practice at their fingertips, how can they be expected to function in a system that demands a delicate balance between the legitimate needs of members and the limited resources of the HMO? They can't be; they have been trained in another system that placed no emphasis on this balance. If they are hired, they will be dysfunctional, rendering service that will be useless at best and disastrous at worst. Departmental morale as a whole will suffer, bringing on many other attendant problems. It is actually much kinder not to hire those who have been steeped in the "bigger is better" mind-set than to hire them and invite trouble for them, the members, and the HMO.

A note before going on to the next section: In HMO departments of mental health I have consulted with whose data indicated poor provider morale, a high in-patient utilization rate, and low member satisfaction, without exception I have observed a predominance of the fee-for-service mentality in the line staff and not infrequently in the director of the department as well. Managerial personnel in these HMOs were, of course, aware that "something" was amiss but were hesitant to intervene because they were not mental health professionals. It is hoped that this book will increase the range of knowledge and confidence in managers such as these and guide them toward instituting early corrective action.

RESUMÉ REVIEW

Resumés are often helpful, but their importance in staff selection should not be overemphasized. Because so few applicants have prior HMO experience, this lack cannot per se be used to eliminate prospective providers.

What kinds of work experience lead to HMO-compatible practice habits? Is there a prototype of mental health service delivery already in existence that incorporates the elements of comprehensiveness and continuity of care, crisis intervention, psychological education, the use of community resources, and almost every other basic concept associated with effective prepaid mental health care? Yes. The principles of community mental health embody all these elements; CMHCs for years have been obligated to deliver very comprehensive services in the face of fixed, cost-contained budgets to mandated populations. That is also what HMOs do. The sources of funding and statutes governing HMO departments of mental health and CMHCs are different, but the concepts and procedural techniques learned in community mental health work can be applied to good advantage in an HMO. If an applicant's resumé shows CMHC experience, look more closely; chances are that a great many vital skills already have been acquired.

Emergency departments are another excellent recruitment source. The HMO is a medical setting in which mental health therapists are all too frequently confronted with multiple crisis situations comparable to those of an emergency department. To function with top efficiency in such "pressure cooker" atmospheres, therapists must possess the following attributes or skills:

- Clinical versatility (being a generalist)

- Skills in rapid assessment and disposition

- Expertise in medical evaluation

- Ability to work as part of a treatment team (of particular importance).

Emergency settings *demand* these attributes. They are the *sine qua non* of a seasoned emergency department staff member and fit in very nicely with HMO work. If the resumé indicates emergency department experience, the applicant should be asked if it was enjoyable. If so, these applicants also should be considered carefully.

What other types of work settings produce therapists whose theoretical sets and practice habits are compatible with the requirements of an HMO department of mental health? Ironically, there seems to be an inverse correlation between the real value of a provider to an HMO and the "professional" status of the provider's previous employment setting. For example, child protective service workers in county social service departments, public health or visiting nurses, psychologists and social workers, and outpatient and inpatient therapists working in county, state, or Veterans Administration mental health settings all enjoy far less "professional" status than do providers in private outpatient and inpatient units or therapists in prestigious university medical centers. This lack of professional status is in reality the lack of social status associated with these settings, which are often low paying, understaffed, and extremely demanding. But it is precisely here that the astute HMO manager or departmental director should step in and take advantage of the training, skills, and motivation of these individuals. They work in systems that demand flexibility and innovativeness, two very important traits to the prepaid sector, with its high ambulatory utilization and limited resources.

DEGREES

When recruiting time comes, a great deal of debate often occurs over what degrees the department's line-providers should have—M.S.W., M.S.N., R.N., M.S., or M.A.? Much of this debate can be eliminated (not to mention the time wasted in the formation of tedious task forces assigned to "study" the question) by employing the concept of role equivalency. What are the required tasks, and what attributes are necessary to accomplish these tasks without regard to specific academic degrees?

When all the professional hocus-pocus is eliminated, the essence of what we do is deliver the "therapeutic conversation." What does this require? By far the majority of ambulatory mental health encounters in any sector require only a finite number of attributes, the most important of which are flexibility and the ability to relate to another person. In other words, can the provider reformulate a treatment plan quickly and imaginatively if the initial formulation is inadequate or inaccurate, and is he or she capable of talking to a so-called patient in an honest and noncondescending manner? These two attributes have nothing to do with degrees, but everything to do with the person. A productive therapeutic conversation is impossible in the face of rigidity and exalted professionalism.

Actually, role equivalency is not a new concept. The day has long passed when community standards and insurance requirements demand that mental health service be delivered by either a psychiatrist or a licensed Ph.D. clinical psychologist. Today, the other specialties mentioned above are all being used in the private, community, and prepaid sectors. However, current reliable data regarding the extent to which mid-level providers are employed in HMO departments of mental health are almost nonexistent (chapter 7, which deals with staffing ratios and mix, lists what current information is available on this subject). Suffice it to say that at present, the HMO recruiter should not be sidetracked into time-consuming, esoteric analyses of the comparative benefits of hiring an M.S.W. as opposed to an M.S.N. or an M.A. as opposed to an M.S. psychologist. The required tasks should be kept in mind, and the person, not the degree, should be the deciding factor in choosing mental health line providers.

A proviso to the above must also be kept in mind. Nonmedical providers (social workers and psychologists) must be medically sophisticated, and medical mid-level providers (bachelor's and master's level nurses) and psychologists must have at least the basic rudiments of social work skills.

For example, although social workers and psychologists cannot prescribe psychotropic medication, they should know the various classes of these drugs along with their dosage range, side effects, and contraindications to prescribing them. They also should be able to clinically evaluate and monitor a member's response to these medications and be ready to alert a physician to any "untoward event" such as a paradoxical response, an allergic response, or obvious member noncompliance with the dosage regimen. The old social worker's or psychologist's saw of "Have you spoken to your doctor about this?" shouldn't be accepted in an HMO.

As for social work skills that should be expected of mid-level medical providers and psychologists, the practitioner should at minimum be able to think collaboratively; that is, what other agency or organization can assist in this treatment situation or even may be essential to its successful resolution? That sort of thought process is second nature to psychiatric social workers, but not necessarily to nurses and psychologists, who often perceive it as a quantum leap in mentation. Nevertheless, such a transition must be made if valuable community resources are to be used. This isn't just a matter of conserving the HMO's limited resources; many cases cannot be brought to a successful termination without the assistance of protective services, shelters for battered women, Alcoholics Anonymous, and similar organizations and agencies.

Another way of approaching this facet of the provider selection process is to apply the concept of clinical versatility. Is the applicant a generalist or someone with a narrow range of clinical expertise? In other words, can the provider be relied upon to function adequately in whatever clinical setting he or she is placed? I remember one nightmare situation in which I had "inherited" the administrative responsibility where case after case went "sour." Why? The answers I received while conducting an on-line investigation were most informative: "Yes, I did notice that the patient was staggering when I tested him, but I'm a psychologist, not a doctor." (The patient had misunderstood the instructions for taking his medication, had grossly overmedicated himself, and had fallen down a flight of stairs after leaving the psychologist's office.) And, "I saw no reason to refer the woman to a shelter . . . she had always been able to handle her husband's outbursts before." (The husband's prior outbursts had almost put the patient in the hospital on several occasions, the one I was following up had finally succeeded—the woman at least should have been given information about shelters for battered women at the beginning of therapy.) If line providers consider themselves specialists and not generalists, then sooner or later they will make these sorts of errors.

Chapter 5
THE DIRECTOR'S ROLE

What should be expected of an HMO mental health director? To answer this question it is necessary to examine the various needs he or she must attempt to satisfy. These needs may be divided into five major categories: (1) member needs, (2) plan needs, (3) mental health staff needs, (4) nonmental health staff needs, and (5) other needs (employers, unions, outside agencies, etc.).

Before discussing these needs in detail, a note of optimism seems appropriate. Those who have previously written on this topic have correctly stressed the difficulty of achieving a functioning balance between forces whose goals often appear to be in conflict. They have nòt, I believe, sufficiently stressed the fact that a great deal of this conflict *is* apparent, and that the HMO provides a matrix in which common interest may replace conflict in addressing the legitimate needs of all parties.

For example, low provider productivity may appear to be in the best interest of the mental health staff unless it is appreciated that one of the quickest ways to experience professional dissatisfaction and burnout is to have so little to do that busywork must be created. Or a union representative may feel that it is in the member's best interests to obtain a three-month mental health leave of absence from work if the representative is not aware of the fact that prolonged leaves of absence potentiate emotional dysfunction and psychoinvalidism. Or, as mentioned in chapter 1, it may appear to be in the HMO's best interest to scrimp in offering ambulatory care until it is recognized that savings of this sort will be far outweighed by costs on the inpatient side.

In the discussions that follow, I will attempt to expand on the theme of common interest replacing conflict.

MEMBER NEEDS

In trying to establish policies and procedures that satisfy the needs of the membership, the departmental director must differentiate between legitimate and nonlegitimate needs. This process of differentiation frequently exposes the director to the charge of being arbitrary, or worse, of being an autocrat. The resultant flak can be extremely unnerving, but it must be worked through because this issue is far too important to be ignored. For example, a plan's marketing brochure may state that members may choose their own providers. This statement is frequently interpreted by HMO members to mean unlimited freedom of choice. They fail to understand that the only system that gives unlimited freedom of provider selection is the "you pay everything out of your own pocket" system. All health insurance contracts place limitations on provider selection. Prepaid contracts merely have more specific limitations than indemnity contracts; that is, the member is limited, except in emergency situations, to care rendered by plan-approved providers. This is a matter of contractual agreement and ideally should not be a point of controversy, but as noted in chapter 3, it all too often causes controversy because of inadequate member orientation.

Legitimate controversy with which the director must deal does, however, arise in the question of choice among approved providers. Not infrequently, a member is evaluated and assigned to a given therapist; a week or even months may pass, whereupon the director is confronted with the member's request for a change of therapist. It is tempting to interpret all of these requests as member "resistance to positive change" and deal with them on the basis of noncompliance, but that won't do. Sometimes the member's dissatisfaction is quite legitimate.

Every request for reassignment must be evaluated, a time-consuming but informative activity. The best approach is to discuss the matter with the therapist first. During this discussion, it often becomes evident that a "mismatch" has occurred and that a reassignment is in order. If nothing conclusive results from this meeting, a half-hour appointment should be scheduled with the member. Frequently, just the fact that someone took the time to listen to a complaint is enough to cause the member to decide to continue with the assigned provider. More important, however, this meeting gives the director a chance for early monitoring of undetected critical situations that could result in legal action. It never pays for a director to become separated from the day-to-day line operations of the department; it is simply a form of practical quality assurance.

The director frequently is called upon to make policy and individual decisions in the thorny issue of member advocacy. At face value, most therapists would consider this a nonissue: "Of course we should act as advocates . . . that's what we've been taught, and it makes sense." Granted, that is what we were taught, and it does make sense; but does it make sense in all circumstances? Does it make sense to continue to extend a member's mental health leave of absence from work if he or she is able to return to work? Does it make sense to support a member's workers compensation claim when it is clear to the therapist that work had nothing to do with the member's difficulties? Does it make sense to help a member avoid the criminal justice system by enfranchising him or her in the mental health system when it is evident that the prosecutor's allegations are true?

Legitimate need can literally act as a clarifying concept here. Not only are the above three situations examples of nonlegitimate member needs but they also represent conspiracy pitfalls for therapists (fraud in the first two examples and potential perjury in the third). The director must constantly bear in mind that whatever goes into the mental health record may well need to be defended in court proceedings other than malpractice.

The point might seem belabored, but the issue is extremely important. It encompasses far more than the average member's misunderstanding of what can realistically be expected from the plan's benefit package. This misunderstanding, based on a lack of information, can be corrected by educating members about what constitutes effective mental health care. The issue referred to here does not emanate from individual misunderstanding, but rather from a global societal distress syndrome.

As the technological revolution accelerates, competition for jobs and demands for increased productivity are becoming harsher and harsher. Workers, whether in manufacturing or service, whether hourly workers or salaried professionals, regard this revolution as extremely threatening. Conflict in the workplace is often a result of this perceived threat, and conflict leads to the search for advocates. This is the point at which the mental health department is often requested to enter the arena, sometimes appropriately, sometimes not.

Unquestionably, unreserved advocacy should be provided in cases in which there is clear-cut evidence of employer abuse or harassment. That's an ethical given. But what about clear-cut evidence of featherbedding or malingering? Historically, this question (as any physician who has done IMO* examinations can attest) unfortunately posed no problem for many fee-for-service psychiatrists: So long as the examination fee was paid,

---

IMO stands for independent medical opinion. These examinations, for determining whether an employee is able to return to work or not, are usually paid for by both the employer and the union.

the excuse was written. This is the ambience in which the HMO mental health provider must attempt to function. The line dividing advocacy and co-conspiracy has become virtually invisible for many members and providers.

Neither the director of mental health nor HMO managers can ignore this issue of nonlegitimate requests (more frequently demands) for inappropriate mental health intervention. It is not only an issue of defrauding an employer or a private or public insurance fund, but is also an issue of correct sociopolitical action. If the technological revolution is to be governed by humane principles, then the voices of its critics should be heard in the areas of conflict and not allowed to opt out into the mental health system and thereby remain silent.

Once determined, these kinds of policy decisions must be communicated by the director to the line providers, who bear the brunt of all members' requests and demands. They must clearly understand the policies, be willing to carry them out, and not succumb to misguided humanitarianism or member harassment (malingerers can expend up to and beyond 10 times the amount of energy required to do their jobs in attempts to avoid those jobs). In-service training sessions during which the entire problem is discussed frankly can be quite helpful here.

The example previously cited of attempting to avoid the criminal justice system by using the mental health department as an advocate need not be a problem for an HMO mental health department. Many HMOs simply avoid this headache by preparing a policy statement to the effect that "court-ordered and defense-requested mental health evaluations are not benefits covered under the contract." This policy, of course, allows for exceptions to be made in those few cases in which the member has a bona fide mental health defense.

However the department proceeds in this matter, the director will still come under fire. If a choice is made to sidestep the issue via the above sort of policy statement, then the court, defense attorneys, involved members, and union representatives will complain of inadequate service delivery. If the issue is tackled head-on by agreeing to do these sorts of evaluations, then pressure from defense attorneys and their member-clients for acceptable findings will be forthcoming, not to mention the drain on departmental resources from hours spent in examinations, depositions, and court appearances.

The need for members to have easy access to a mental health provider is one of the few issues on which the director encounters general agreement. Even an overextended mental health staff would agree in principle that quick access to the system is necessary for the delivery of high quality care. Immediate access reduces the length and severity of emotional distress, hospital bed days, days missed from work, and the amount of sick benefits paid out.

The topic of accessibility of service was covered in chapter 2 insofar as its importance and techniques to bring it about are concerned. What interests us here is the director's role in maintaining this essential characteristic of a high-quality, cost-effective system once it is established. All systems tend to experience a certain amount of "drift" from the optimum unless they are monitored, and mental health is no exception. Here, departure from the ideal usually appears as a gradual lengthening of access time for evaluating members in crisis because of an increasing member-to-staff ratio that causes a lowering of staff morale (line providers who are overworked will merely redefine crisis as urgent or even routine). This is an area in which the director must maintain a vigilant but diplomatic eye. The task of monitoring access should not be delegated; as in the investigation of requests for therapist reassignment, it is a form of practical quality assurance. Watching the member-to-staff ratio, checking the number of available open slots in the departmental schedule, and—most important—sensing morale by spending an adequate amount of time with staff are useful monitoring procedures for a director who is determined to keep access time within acceptable limits.

PLAN NEEDS

Probably more than any other service, mental health care represents a dilemma to HMO managers. Bluntly stated, they often don't have the vaguest idea of what's really going on in the department, but their mandate or need is to know. In doing mental health consultations around the country, I have noted that managerial attempts to resolve this dilemma usually fall into one of two categories, both counterproductive: The manager, in lieu of information, either tries to dictate departmental policy and procedure or accepts unquestioningly whatever policies, procedures, and outcomes the department generates. As mentioned in chapter 1, the genesis of this managerial bind lies in the mistaken assumption that mental health work is almost totally nonquantifiable and therefore is not open to the kinds of administrative review and critique to which other departments are subjected.

It is here that the departmental director has an opportunity to play an invaluable role. He or she can teach managerial personnel the basics of good HMO mental health policies, procedures, and service delivery. Once this knowledge is imparted, then rational dialogue can take place regarding such plan concerns as benefit design, quality of service, costs, and the satisfaction level of members, employers, unions, and state and federal regulatory agencies. Actually, these are not just plan concerns; they vitally affect all parties involved in the design, marketing, purchase, and delivery of prepaid mental health services. Again, a spirit of cooperation in sharing information is the ideal that both the director and managerial personnel should strive to implement.

Monthly meetings between the departmental director and key managers should be scheduled. These meetings provide not only an educational opportunity but also an excellent forum for managerial monitoring and input. For example, the time could be used to review the previous month's utilization data and to discuss member complaints, enrollment figures, hiring of new providers, and the need for new programs.

The premise underlying this interchange between director and management is that areas of legitimate managerial input can be delineated in mental health, but only if management clearly understands the essential elements of mental health policy/procedure and service delivery. If these elements are understood, then the HMO manager can effectively approach the task of evaluation and goal setting and provide guidelines for overall departmental functioning without encroaching on the turf of the mental health professional.

Although the specifics of benefit design, quality assurance, policy and procedure development, and cost of service will be dealt with in other chapters, it is worthwhile to pause and examine a troublesome issue that is too often viewed by plan management as a need: providing consultation and therapy to plan employees who are also plan members. From the plan's perspective, it makes sense to provide this service to its employee. It saves money on outside referrals, and in some cases (not many, fortunately), it serves to control troublesome, dissatisfied employees. But cost savings and expediency do not outweigh the problems this arrangement creates. Even at best, when the disturbance is mild and transient, and responds well to therapy, there remains a residuum of discomfort on the part of both provider and employee. Mixing the roles of coworker and therapist causes strain. At worst, when employees have grievances—founded or unfounded— against the plan, the mental health department is placed in the untenable position of being advocate to opposing parties. The drain on departmental resources and the potential of being placed in a conflict-of-interest situation are not conducive to efficient departmental operations and high plan morale. It is incumbent upon the director to point out this potential pitfall to management. Considerable effort may have to be expended in order to bring about a change in managerial thinking, but it is time well spent. In the long run, it is better to make the outside referral and pay the cost for plan employees than to be in a double bind that may have unforseen legal consequences.

MENTAL HEALTH STAFF NEEDS

In a recent article, Berman and McLaughlin listed the needs of mental health staff members as " . . . good compensation; emphasis on quality, not productivity; more administrative and supervision time; the opportunity to do long-term psychotherapy; and interdisciplinary equality".[5] Although not totally exhaustive, the list sums up the matter pretty well.

Where should the mental health director stand in regard to staff needs? Unfortunately, the answer is right in the middle of the fray. Janus-like, the director has one face turned toward management and one toward the department's providers—a potentially schizophrenogenic position. The department's success or failure depends in great measure (the larger the department the more this applies) on the director's "style of leadership"—but what style works best? In actuality, no one particular style works better than any other. I know of several effective, smooth-running departments in which democracy reigns; on the other hand, I am also aware of top-notch departments of mental health in which the smell of autocracy cannot be missed.

The common factor in all successful departments is the lack of ambiguity; everyone is clear about how power is deployed, and the rules of the game are known. My own style might be characterized as laissez faire with teeth. I make sure that departmental policies and procedures are known to all staff members and I keep myself unobtrusively available to them for consultation, but woe to the one who blunders because of negligence! I should also add that I pay my providers about 10 percent more than the going rate in the area.

Good compensation, as Berman and McLaughlin

indicated, is understandably an important issue with staff. Provider salaries and benefits should be competitive plus. Where is cost containment, you say? If an HMO of 40,000 has been experiencing mental health inpatient costs of more than $400,000 per year but is aiming at a cost of one-third that figure, then an extra $15,000 to $20,000 divided among six or seven providers is not a significant expense when compared to its incentive value. Each well-spent dollar on the ambulatory side will save many dollars on the inpatient side.

However, convincing top management of the wisdom of this expenditure is frequently difficult when graduating psychiatric social workers and master's level psychologists can by hired at between $18,000 and $19,000 a year. It is necessary for the director to use experience in delivering mental health service to educate management. For example, the director must demonstrate that the $8,000 to $12,000 saved by hiring a "greenhorn" will be more than offset by the hours of costly teaching and supervision this person will require and by the dollars wasted in unnecessary hospitalizations due to the person's inability to handle difficult cases. The director also must point out to management that because HMO mental health work is considerably more stressful than traditional fee-for-service work, it is worth a premium salary and benefits. This is especially true in the present phase of HMO development, when a great deal of provider time must be spent in correcting unrealistic member expectations regarding their actual entitlement.

Unless the line providers' compensation is satisfactory (plus a margin to cover the stress factor), all parties involved in the prepaid transaction will suffer. First of all, the provider will experience lowered morale, which will give rise to far-reaching and *very* detrimental consequences:

1. The department's turnover rate will be high, with a concomitant decrease in continuity of care for members.

2. Members will receive less than enthusiastic, first-rate service, and the HMO's public relations and enrollment figure will suffer.

3. The hospitalization rate will increase because the therapists lack the spirit necessary to stay on top of a case that is not going well.

4. The likelihood of member suicide will increase for the same reason that the hospitalization rate increases.

5. The chance of the plan's being successfully sued for malpractice will rise because a decrease in quality of service is accompanied by an increased risk of "therapeutic misadventure."

6. The specter of provider unionization becomes larger when morale among staff is generally low.

Although compensation is extremely important and should never be overlooked, it is not *only* a matter of money (the index of avarice is no higher in a mental health department than in any other department). In point of fact, any or all of the above-listed negative consequences are more likely to occur whenever overall staff morale is lowered for a significant period of time for whatever reason. This gives the director, who is the staff's primary advocate and arbiter, ample motivation to address staff needs as they arise and not wait until they are overwhelming.

The debate about quality versus productivity is a multifaceted issue, but it is frequently more related to the issue of long-term versus short-term therapy than to the matter of quality per se. Here, as in so many areas of HMO mental health, an ounce of foresight will prevent a ton of dispute: Hire only those providers who are comfortable with and competent in delivering short-term therapy. If this is done, the debate can then advance to a rational form because all parties are using the same language (there are as many dialects of "therapese" as there are schools of therapy). If this is not done, then hours—even weeks—of valuable time will be wasted in contention regarding quality when the underlying theme is really the orientation to long-term therapy.

Disputes over quality versus productivity will occur even when the staff is hand-picked and in mutual agreement with the precepts of prepaid mental health service delivery. However, here the operational issues at point are manageable: administrative versus clinical time, and how many clinical encounters are required per week or month. Framed in those terms, the matter of quality and productivity can be resolved to the satisfaction of both staff and plan by the director's input and guidance.

Whether or not a department should provide time for formal supervision of line therapists is an issue that is still debated in many HMOs, although the majority of plans probably come down on the side of supervision. Even those plans that do not set aside time for supervision still provide the equivalent de facto via informal or "hallway" consultation with peers, unit directors, or the departmental director. Feedback from other clinicians is essential and not a subject for plan-prescribed mandates. The question is not whether this feedback should or should not take place, but whether it should be formalized and the required time reimbursed. Those directors who do not provide formal supervisory hours argue that the HMO is not a training center and that the members' premiums are paid for professionals who are capable of practicing independently. They point out that the prepaid sector is in competition with a system (fee-for-service medicine) that provides no compensation for supervisory time and conference time; in other words, HMOs are competing against a "no work, no pay" adversary.

I do not agree with this stand. Time should be allotted for supervision and also for continued training in the form of conferences and workshops. Supervisory time is usually scheduled by two methods. The first, which I prefer, is to integrate supervision into a weekly staff meeting, thereby gaining several advantages. If supervision is handled in this manner, much like "chart rounds" on a medical or surgical ward, then problem case management is beneficially augmented by input from the entire staff and not just one supervisor. Other advantages to this method are:

- Flexibility (Supervisory time can be expanded or contracted as needed within the limits of the staff meeting so that all cases are covered, but no time is wasted.)

- Satisfaction of the quality assurance requirement of peer review (Therefore, this part of the staff meeting should be documented.)

- Acquainting all staff members with current difficult cases in which they might be called upon to intervene either as walk-ins or while on call.

■ Generating an increased sense of esprit de corps in the department via the process of collegial problem solving.

■ Education (The method of group supervision serves as a teaching forum for each staff provider.)

The other, more formal method of providing supervision is to schedule each therapist for a certain number of hours per month of individual supervision with his or her unit director or the departmental director. This would amount to an hour of one-to-one supervision every one to two weeks. At first glance, this may not seem to be excessive, but it can involve up to a day a week of a supervisor's time for each seven providers in the department. This is a significant expenditure of time. In short, although individual supervision is more traditional than group supervision, it is time consuming and has few of the special advantages of group supervision.

Whatever system of supervision is chosen for the department, the value of informal "hallway" consultation should never be overlooked. From departmental director to mental health assistant, each staff member is an integral part of the treatment team and can contribute to treatment regardless of where this contribution takes place. Therefore, the director should not only encourage informal consultations among staff but must set an example by being available for this sort of supervision.

The matter of paid time to attend HMO conferences and workshops involves even more controversy than paid supervisory time. Most plans will pay for senior mental health staff members to attend a conference, but it is much more difficult to obtain plan approval (and money) for line providers to attend. The same arguments that are used against paid supervisory time are mobilized against paid educational time. In my opinion, this is another example of misguided managerial parsimony. Not only do conferences impart useful information but they also reduce professional isolation, reaffirm professional identity, and serve as an intellectual stimulant that can promote new, creative ideas and programs in the department. In the role of staff advocate, the departmental director should lobby for paid educational time as a benefit for all mental health staff members. The amount of time off and the percentage of the conference or workshop that is paid for can vary with length of service or rank in the department, but the benefit should be universal.

Interdisciplinary equality, which Berman and McLaughlin referred to, is also a legitimate staff need. This topic was covered as role equivalency in the section on degrees in chapter 4, but is worthy of more comment. The alternative to interdisciplinary equality is an artificial and counterproductive interdisciplinary snobbery with roots in traditional, rigid professionalism. The burgeoning prepaid mental health sector has no place for this attitude; it undermines staff morale and leads to petty squabbling and lasting resentment among providers.

The acid test of value in a department is whether or not a therapist can accomplish the required task. Using this yardstick, along with length of service in the organization and years of experience in the field, it is possible to construct a salary scale that reflects a provider's value to the plan. Again, it is up to departmental directors, especially if they are psychiatrists, to set this tone of egalitarianism in the department. This does not mean that they should abandon their administrative authority (that would lead to chaos), but it does mean that they should eschew behaviors based on an appeal to the authority of academic degrees rather than ability.

NONMENTAL HEALTH STAFF NEEDS

Departments of mental health have the tendency to become insular, to lose effective working contact with other services in the HMO. The primary causes of this schism arise in the prevalent and long-standing attitudes of other medical specialists toward mental health and in the mental health department's reaction to these attitudes. Bluntly stated, providers in other specialties are often of the opinion that the only accomplishment of the mental health service is to talk in circles. The image of the ineffectual, flimflamming psychiatrist has become a stereotype in our culture. As a reaction to this, mental health workers frequently become defensive and obscure in their communication with physician specialists, creating a far from ideal milieu in which to deliver comprehensive, managed health care delivery.

The earliest historical root of this misunderstanding in the United States dates back to the second half of the nineteenth century in the adversarial relationship between the American Medical Association (AMA) and the Association of Medical Superintendents of American Institutions for the Insane (later to become the American Psychiatric Association). The AMA became aware that European medical schools were developing departments of psychological medicine in an attempt to move mental health practice into the mainstream of medicine. This integration appeared to be worthwhile to the AMA, inasmuch as mental health service delivery in this country had developed in relative isolation from the rest of medicine. Starting in 1868, the AMA sent delegates to the yearly conference of the medical superintendents group to formally propose a merger, but the efforts were rebuffed repeatedly for several years. The superintendents were undoubtedly fearful of what is known today as an "unfriendly merger." Resistance to a closer relationship between the two associations was "diplomatically" verbalized by the medical superintendents' president at the 1869 meeting as follows:

> I am sure the whole medical profession must sympathize deeply with the great and laudable purposes of the American Medical Association, and I am confident none more so than the members of this body. Yet for various reasons—good and sufficient as we believe them—we think now, as we have always thought, that it is best for us, and the cause we represent, that we should retain our distinct and separate organization.[6]

And that was that. This rejection of a merger, "good and sufficient" as it may have been, could not have resulted in anything but increased antagonism toward and suspicion of mental health by medical practitioners and further isolation of the field from mainstream medicine.

A less remote, and still ongoing, cause of medicine's perplexed attitude toward mental health can be traced back to the heyday of analytically oriented fee-for-service practice. To illustrate, let's say that a conscientious but overworked internist in 1955 referred a recently diagnosed diabetic patient for a psychiatric consultation. The patient is functioning fairly well, but the internist had read a journal article listing the potential benefits of a counseling session in helping diabetics adjust to their condition. The internist calls the psychiatrist for some feedback on the case (an evaluation summary was never sent), but what does he hear? Probably one of the following responses:

- A long and very confusing monologue, couched in what sounds like Greek and Latin words of questionable scientific veracity, on unconscious self-destructive impulses. The bottom line of this "consultation" is that the diabetic patient is *much* sicker than was ever imagined and has now embarked upon a long course of psychoanalysis.

- A slightly haughty refusal to discuss the case because of a potential breach of confidentiality. The bottom line of this "consultation" is the same as the previous one.

Could anything be better designed to create suspicion and animosity among the providers of nonmental health care?

In order for HMO members to receive first-class, comprehensive care, the staffs of *all* departments not only should have mutual respect for one another but also should understand and respond effectively to one another's needs in delivering service. What are the needs of nonmental health providers with respect to mental health? Although there are other related and nonrelated issues, easy access and practical advice top the list in importance by a significant margin.

Easy access means that a referral from internal medicine, surgery, pediatrics, or other departments will be seen by a mental health provider as soon as necessary with an absolute minimum of cumbersome clerical procedures. In operational terms, this means that a nonmental health provider who has a member "falling apart" during an office visit can walk that member down to the mental health department with the assurance that an evaluation will be completed within the hour. Expectations of this sort place a strain on the department, but are quite legitimate and should be met. After all, doesn't the mental health department expect internal medicine to respond immediately to a possible acute myocardial infarction occurring in mental health? Whoever heads the department, physician or not, should carefully draw up policies and procedures for expeditiously processing these internal referrals and should alert the staff to their importance. Not all internal referrals will have to be seen so quickly, but it is much wiser to be available and accept a few inappropriate referrals than to risk becoming inapproachable. The resulting interdepartmental harmony will more than offset any wasted time.

Simple and clear suggestions or instructions should be easily attainable by nonmental health providers on how they should manage patients who manifest emotional problems. Also, the mental health department must anticipate problems that providers in other departments might encounter with joint cases —for example, warning them about possible side effects of psychotropic medication and alerting them to member noncompliance that might have a negative impact on case management.

Because the mental health department must be viewed by other providers as approachable, it must remain visible. One of the most efficient techniques for maintaining a high profile is to conduct in-service training sessions. The departmental director should consider this educational effort as having high priority and not delegate it.

Interdepartmental in-service sessions are reciprocal in terms of information flow; that is, they teach basic mental health skills and also give valuable feedback to mental health providers. This feedback is often voiced in the form of complaints, but that's fine —don't become defensive. Encourage providers in other departments to say whatever they will. This is one of the best barometers for monitoring the interdepartmental "atmosphere."

An in-service training program need not be an elaborate endeavor; one 45-minute session per month is sufficient. Topics should include identification and early referral of high-risk members, basic crisis intervention techniques, simple and safe use of psychotropic medication with guidelines for assessment of side effects, and evaluation of suicide potential. Training sessions of this sort maximize the therapeutic skills of providers in all departments and assist in bringing about an integrated system of delivery with minimal interdepartmental friction.

OTHER NEEDS

In concluding this examination of the role of the departmental director, let us look at the needs of those interests outside the HMO. These outside interests include employers, union and employee assistance program representatives, attorneys, other insurance companies, medical providers not associated with the HMO, and agencies such as social service departments, courts, and police departments. The theme that connects these interests is their desire for mental health information about members.

A word of caution here: Before any information is released, verbal or written, the request should be carefully evaluated for appropriateness. Who wants the information? Why do they want it? Next, a release of information form should be executed by the member or the member's legal guardian. The matter of information release is far too important to leave to chance. There must be a fail-safe procedure in place for validating the authenticity and appropriateness of the release of information request and recording the release permission.

A safeguard in the matter of confidentiality is the proper design of the release of information form. It should have a blank for the specific type of information to be released with the written proviso, "...including any drug and/or alcohol abuse information and/or any mental health information," and another blank for the purpose and need for such disclosure. But whatever form is chosen, it should be reviewed carefully by the HMO's legal counsel.

Another cautionary note: Unless the request specifies "a complete narrative," be parsimonious. Most requests from employers, unions, and insurance companies can be satisfied by listing the dates of service, diagnosis, and anticipated lengths of leaves of absence.

Release of full information to other medical providers need not be questioned if the above cautionary procedures have been observed; that is simply good, standard medical practice. However, problems arise when requests for clinical information come from those whose goal is something other than providing health care service. For example, employers or their representatives sometimes will ask for information about a member with no hidden disciplinary agenda in mind; they are merely interested in the employee's progress. Such situations require diplomacy, especially if the request is made by telephone. There is a temptation to cooperate and "give them a little information," but this must be resisted as being very unwise. It is better to briefly but politely explain the rules governing confidentiality, and to indicate that the caller might want to ask the employee to sign a release of information form. In most cases, that is the end of the matter.

Courts and police departments represent a special situation in terms of information release—not special privilege (they have to abide by the rules of confidentiality also) but special pressure. Not infrequently, a court representative or police officer will demand access to a member's chart without a signed release of information form. The HMO is on firm ground if it takes the position of "If there is no signed release, then there must be a subpoena." Also, the subpoena must be bona fide. I remember one case in which a police officer/HMO member was under investigation by a police internal review board for a very serious matter. Officers representing the review board presented what they claimed was a subpoena and demanded the chart. On close inspection, however, the document turned out to be an internal subpoena valid only within the police department itself. It is cases like this one that argue for the departmental director having easy access to the HMO's legal counsel.

Chapter 6
CHOOSING A DIRECTOR

One decision that must be made in the earliest or prerecruitment phase of the process of choosing a departmental director is: Should the departmental head be a psychiatrist or a nonpsychiatrist? This is not such a clear-cut matter as it might appear at first glance. Nothing inherent in the duties of a mental health departmental director demands that the position be filled by a psychiatrist. Most community mental health centers in the United States (more than 1,500 of them) are directed by nonpsychiatrists. Also, psychiatrists are expensive. The HMO will spend at least twice as much in salary and benefits for a psychiatrist as for a nonpsychiatrist.

Why, then, are most HMO departments of mental health directed by psychiatrists? In many instances, the answer to this question is a combination of precedence and expediency. For example, the incorporated medical groups that provide service to group model HMOs are traditionally administered on a departmental basis by physician-managers; that is, there is a surgeon for surgery, a pediatrician for pediatrics, and a psychiatrist for mental health. The precedent of a psychiatrist-director has been set in these groups, and deviation from this policy would meet with marked resistance. It's a matter of guarding professional turf. The situation in staff model HMOs, especially in older plans, is much the same as in group models; at the time these departments were organized, there seemed to be no other choice than a psychiatrist-director.

Are there advantages in choosing a psychiatrist rather than, say, a Ph.D. psychologist or medical social worker to head the department? In my view, the major advantage psychiatrists have is versatility. Not only can they manage a department and provide direct service but their degree allows them to perform psychiatric medical evaluations, write prescriptions, and last but not least, interact on a peer basis with other physicians inside and outside the HMO. The value of the functions of psychiatric medical assessment and prescription writing should not be underestimated; they are necessary and will, therefore, have to be paid for in one way or another.

A further note on the necessity of physician input to the department: As indicated, even if a department is organized without a psychiatrist as director, funds will still need to be allocated for physician coverage. This can be done in two ways. Either a liaison-consultation model is developed in which internists or family practitioners are used for medical assessments and prescription writing or a psychiatrist (more than one if the HMO has a large enrollment) is used as a specialized line provider—that is, not as a general psychotherapist.

Unless there are persuasive reasons to do otherwise, my advice to managers is to come down on the side of a psychiatrist-director, but to be very careful in the final selection process to assure HMO compatibility. The issue of HMO compatibility has already been discussed in chapter 4, and its importance cannot be overemphasized. The criteria discussed in chapter 4 for the selection of line providers are twice as important when selecting a departmental director. Choosing an inappropriate line provider is, after all, only a potential disaster, but a director who is incompatible with an HMO setting is an assured catastrophe.

Above and beyond being knowledgeable in and comfortable with the style of practice required in an HMO, what work experience should the prospective director have? The person applying for the position should have at least some prior administrative experience, although he or she need not have been officially designated as a chief, director, or coordinator. The important element here is that there was exposure to, success in, and enjoyment of mental health administrative tasks such as supervising other therapists, allocating personnel, budgeting, and scheduling or coordinating service with other departments or agencies.

The issue of the applicant's capacity for "enjoyment" of his or her job is important. Although most theories of personnel selection would probably not give much credence to the rather nebulous characteristic of "a sense of enthusiasm or excitement about a task," the prepaid sector may provide an exception to the usefulness of this measure of commitment. It is a new field, pioneering in some ways, and not without a sense of mission. The term "true believer" has been applied to those who believe that the HMO movement, with its emphasis on primary prevention and integrated, comprehensive care, represents a health care delivery system that is not only operationally superior but ethically superior as well. I see nothing wrong with being enthusiastic, even to the point of sensing a mission, about developing an alternative health care system in the United States. As indicated in chapter 5, the role of director of mental health in an HMO involves the skillful juggling of what sometimes appears to be impossible and contradictory demands. A little enthusiasm can be very helpful in dealing with the impossible. So if the applicant demonstrates a "gung-ho" attitude, don't be put off; such an attitude might not be measurable on a personnel selection scale, but it nevertheless may be the earmark of a winner in terms of the HMO's managerial needs.

Chapter 7
STAFFING RATIOS AND STAFF MIX

Very little information is available to HMO managers regarding the related topics of staffing ratios and staff mix. There is certainly no data bank or organized body of technical literature to which a manager can turn in attempting to resolve even the most simple issues in these areas. The significant usable literature that defines appropriate staff size and type is based on surveys of existing plans and can be covered with two references: The national HMO mental health survey published in December 1986[2] and Coleman and Kaminsky's chapter on mental health program planning in volume 4 of *Ambulatory Care Systems.*[7]

I will briefly review the findings of these studies, which reflect national averages, and then make suggestions as to what I think would be a realistic approach to setting staff numbers and types.

Variability seems to be the common denominator in the data from these studies (table 7-1).

Table 7-1.
Range of Providers-to-Enrollees Ratios

	Coleman et al[7]	National HMO Survey[2]
Total providers to enrollees	1:3,000 to 1:30,000	1:1,600 to 1:23,000
Psychiatrists to enrollees	1:6,000 to 1:40,000	1:6,000 to 1:104,000
Psychologists to enrollees	1:13,000 to 1:90,000	1:2,500 to 1:200,000
Social workers to enrollees	1:7,900 to 1:26,600	1:3,600 to 1:93,000
Psychiatric nurses to enrollees	————————	1:15,000 to 1:200,000

In fact, a more accurate description of these data would be increasing variability over time. Variability may well be the one aspect of HMO mental health service about which there is total agreement. "There appears to be no fixed set of rules associated with how the mental health services of prepaid group practice plans arrange staffing patterns . . ." and ". . . there is no rational approach as to the division of labor among these major therapeutic disciplines."[7] "Certainly there is no aspect of the medical care delivery system in health maintenance organizations that creates more confusion and diversity than the delivery of mental health services."[5]

Explanations for this diversity are themselves quite variable:

1. Different plans offer different levels of service.

2. Different plans enroll populations with diverse patterns of utilization.

3. Prepaid mental health care is a new field and has not clearly defined the roles of its professionals.

Regardless of the causes, the HMO mental health care field seems to be a long way from any consensus as to how many and what kind of providers to use. However, it should be noted that the smallest variance over time shown in table 7-1 is for the range of total providers to enrollees ratio. This ratio, more than any other, is governed by reality rather than theoretical demands. This, of course, is only common sense; a provider can be expected to render service to only so many enrollees, and that number is relatively independent of levels of service, differences in patterns of utilization, or age of the field.

TOTAL PROVIDERS-TO-ENROLLEES RATIO

The ratio of total providers to enrollees is the one I examine first when consulting with plans regarding their staffing patterns; more than any other staffing ratio, it reveals how efficiently the department is using clinical personnel. For example, if I see a ratio of 1:1,600, I know without doubt that the department is grossly overstaffed, and that regardless of the inpatient utilization rate, money is being thrown away. (As an aside, overstaffed departments do not tend to generate low hospital bed days; one wonders what they do with their time.) On the other hand, when I see a ratio of 1:30,000, I start looking for the bullwhips and leg irons. Having worked in a setting with a similar ratio, I can attest that the staff was, to put it euphemistically, kept very busy. (As another aside, understaffed departments do occasionally generate very low hospital bed days; in these instances, how the staff spends its time is no mystery.)

The most recent national HMO mental health survey reported some revealing conclusions regarding the relationship between "over- and understaffing" and inpatient utilization:

> It was found that plans with hospital bed days below 30.4 (the national average for group and staff model plans) had an average overall provider ratio of 1:8,506, while those plans with hospital bed days above 30.4 had an average overall provider ratio of 1:5,803. In other words, the more providers, the higher the hospital bed days! This phenomenon seems to demonstrate some combination of Parkinson's Law and the Law of Diminishing Returns, or a shift in focus from utilization goals to a focus on "work load" in some plans. It is noteworthy that the plan with the lowest hospital bed days (2.24) had the leanest overall provider ratio (1:22,727).[2]

Findings of this sort might lead a cynic to conclude that the best policy would be to fire all mental health providers and anticipate that inpatient utilization would drop to zero.

How do these skewed staffing ratios, either over- or

understaffing, come about? The first example, over-staffing, is usually the result of uninformed managers and ambitious directors. Empire building is not limited to field marshals. Some mental health directors like nothing better than to be overstaffed; it gives them a sense of power. They justify their misallocation of personnel by pointing to the fee-for-service work the department does or by citing data from similarly mismanaged departments. If challenged, they respond by raising the specters of malpractice suits, member suicide, and staff burnout. Because most HMO managers have neither hands-on experience in mental health work nor data to support their intuition, they feel compelled to accept the mental health director's demands.

The other extreme, understaffing, is usually caused by inappropriate parsimony and procrastination, both traits reflecting true managerial ineptness. Mental health is in general the last to receive and the first to lose in budgeting; this tendency to undervalue is only accentuated in plans that scrimp in their number of providers. They start by understaffing and then delay adding new providers as the membership increases, even when the need for more staff is evident. When translated into policy, frugality of this sort is very shortsighted; the resulting low provider morale causes untold problems for the plan, the department, and the enrollees (see chapter 5).

What total providers-to-enrollees ratio would allow a mental health department to function with therapeutic efficacy, providing satisfaction to subscribers at acceptable cost? The ratio of 1:7,000 is close to ideal, as the following general example will demonstrate:

HMO X has an enrollment of 50,000. In any given year, about 2,500 members (5 percent) will receive mental health service. The average number of individual "50-minute-hour" sessions generated by this group would be six. Therefore, if only traditional individual therapy were offered, 15,000 hours of provider time would be needed to serve this group. If group therapy is added, then the time requirement will be lower; that is, as noted in chapter 3, a savings in clinical provider time of 58 percent per case can be achieved by using group therapy. If 30 percent of the 2,500 members are treated in groups, then, the required provider hours will be reduced to 12,390. But not all the remaining cases have to be scheduled for an hour; 35 percent or more of them could be scheduled for six half-hour sessions, thus reducing the total number of therapy hours required to 10,552.

How many providers will be required to render the 10,552 hours of therapy? If we assume a 40-hour work week, a 48-week work year (three weeks vacation and one week educational leave), and 80 percent clinical time, then each provider will have 1,536 hours per year available for therapy. Therefore:

$$
\begin{aligned}
\text{Number of full-time equivalent providers required} &= \frac{\text{Number of total therapy hours required per year}}{\text{Number of hours each provider has available for therapy per year}} \\[1em]
&= \frac{10{,}552}{1{,}536} \\[1em]
&= 6.86 \cong 7.0
\end{aligned}
$$

And:

$$
\text{Total providers-to-enrollees ratio} = \frac{\text{Number of enrollees in HMO X}}{\text{Number of FTE providers required}}
$$

$$\text{Total providers-to-enrollees ratio} \left\{ \begin{array}{l} = \dfrac{50,000}{7.0} \\[2ex] = 1{:}7{,}143 \cong 1{:}7{,}000 \end{array} \right.$$

In reviewing this example, it is clear that even if HMOs offered nothing but traditional individual 50-minute-hour psychotherapy, they would still require a total providers-to-enrollees ratio of only about 1:5,000. Any plan with a ratio of 1:6,000 or less should reevaluate its staffing needs, because in all likelihood clinical personnel are not being used to the best advantage. An exception to this is found in departments that have combined mental health and substance abuse services; in these instances, a ratio of 1:5,500 to 1:6,000 is appropriate in view of the increased demand for service.

The 1:7,000 ratio can, of course, be stretched by increasing the percent group therapy (up to 40 percent or more of a plan's caseload can be seen in groups), and/or increasing the percent of half-hour sessions. These maneuvers can be accomplished without sacrificing quality or adding to hospital bed days. The figure suggested allows for a steady flow of work with a more than ample reserve capacity for handling emergencies or other unexpected events.

Table 7-2 can be used as a guide for determining overall mental health and mental health plus substance abuse staffing requirements in HMOs of various sizes.

Two last points regarding the total providers-to-enrollees ratio: Despite a range of 1:1,600 to 1:23,000 (Table 7-1), the 1986 national HMO average for staff and group models was 1:7,521 (Table 7-3). Evidently, the inherent realistic demands of prepaid mental

Table 7-2.
Guide for Determining Required Number of Providers

Membership (in 000s)	No. of Providers for Mental Health Service+	No. of Providers for Mental Health and Substance Abuse Service⁰
10	1.5⊕	2.0
20	3.0	4.0
30	4.5	5.5
40	6.0	7.5
50	7.5	9.5
60	9.0	11.0
70	10.0	13.0
80	11.5	15.0
90	13.0	16.5
100	14.5	18.5
110	16.0	21.0
120	17.5	22.0
130	19.0	24.0
140	20.0	25.5
150	21.5	27.5
160	23.0	29.5

+ = Ratio of 1:7,000
0 = Ratio of 1:5,500
⊕ = All numbers rounded up to nearest 0.5 providers

health care have had an influence on the industry's overall staffing decisions. Also, it should be noted that my overall suggested ratio of 1:7,000 is for psychotherapists—that is, line- or mid-level providers—and is not meant to include psychiatrists. The issue of psychiatrist staffing ratios will be addressed in the following section.

PSYCHIATRIST STAFFING

The number of psychiatrists needed for a properly functioning HMO department of mental health is truly a controversial issue.

The data cited in Tables 7-1 and 7-3 are interesting but not very helpful in deciding this issue, inasmuch as they list only the range and national average number of psychiatrists in staff and group model HMOs and not how this type of professional is used. In order to calculate "how many," we first need to know "for what purpose." Two methods can be used to approach the decision of how many psychiatrists are needed:

■ Develop a department with a psychiatrist-director

■ Develop a department in which psychiatrists are used only as medical subspecialists.

In many ways, the first method is preferable because it avoids the criticism of the American Psychiatric Association and other psychiatric professional associations that have stated that psychiatric services in HMOs, like other psychiatric services, require psychiatric leadership.[8] Also, this method capitalizes on the versatility of the psychiatrist (see chapter 6). However, if the route of psychiatrist-director is chosen, then that individual's duties must be specifically delineated in order to determine the required staffing. It is here that marked differences in practice and opinion occur.

My consulting experience has taught me that a large number of psychiatric directors function as general psychotherapists in addition to doing medical-psychiatric evaluations, writing prescriptions, and doing hospital and managerial work. They spend a great deal of time delivering the "therapeutic conversation" via the 50-minute hour. This is a *very cost-ineffective* use of psychiatric time that has not escaped jovial comment in the literature:

> Let's talk about the role definition of a psychiatrist in an HMO. Psychiatrists don't want to hear this, that's for sure. I see a psychiatrist as a physician-manager and not as a psychotherapist. Their job, as far as I'm concerned, is primarily to treat biologically based mental illness and to behaviorally and administratively manage those patients with significant character disorders. I think most psychiatrists were trained to believe that the most sophisticated skill was doing long-term analytically oriented psychotherapy. At least I was when I was trained, but things seem to be changing. Psychotherapist is not the role I see psychiatrists playing in the HMO. There is a cartoon that I love to share with any psychiatrist I'm recruiting. It's a picture of an obviously obese patient talking with a physician and the physician is saying to the patient, "Mr. Brown, it's really very simple; if it tastes good, spit it out." That's the equivalent of what I say to our psychiatrists: If you see a patient who looks like a great opportunity for psychotherapy, get him out, he goes to a psychotherapist. I see the HMO psychiatrist more and more moving toward a physician-manager role.[9]

I feel that $70,000 to $100,000 a year is a bit steep for a psychotherapist, but if psychiatrists don't provide psychotherapy, what are they to do? It is my opinion that their major duties, aside from treating hospitalized members and performing general administration tasks, should be doing medical psychiatric evaluations and prescription writing. These duties require some explication. Medical-psychiatric evaluations include:

■ Evaluation of members whose medical status is unclear

■ Evaluation of members whose cases might have legal or medicolegal consequences

■ Evaluation of members who are considered to be potentially dangerous

■ Evaluation of members who have serious complaints about the mental health services they or their families have received

■ Evaluation of any member specifically referred to the psychiatrist by another mental health or nonmental health provider within the HMO.

Prescription writing involves not only the initial face-to-face evaluation for psychotropic medication but also follow-up visits with the member for the purpose of judging response; monitoring progress; deciding when to adjust, change, or discontinue medication; and checking for and treating side effects.

How much time do these tasks require? Again, there will be considerable disagreement, especially among psychiatrists, with my stance on this question. Opposition from my colleagues is understandable because I maintain that the prepaid sector can reduce its average number of psychiatrists by 40 percent or more.

It has been estimated that about a third of the HMO members who receive mental health service will require psychiatric attention.[10] This would mean that in the previous example of HMO X, 833 members would need to see a psychiatrist at least once during the year (5 percent of 50,000 members, or 2,500, would require mental health services, and 33 percent of those individuals, or 833, would see a psychiatrist).

My experience leads me to agree with this one-third figure, but a membership figure is not hours. How many psychiatric hours will these 833 members consume in a year? I maintain that 960 hours (0.5 FTE) would suffice to accomplish the task and leave a significant block of time as a reserve. I have observed an interesting relationship between HMO size and the number of FTE psychiatrists required to render ambulatory clinical service. If one were to take the number of HMO enrollees and place a decimal in front of that figure, the result would be the correct staffing for psychiatrists doing ambulatory clinical work. For example, an HMO with 30,000 members would require 0.3 FTE psychiatrists, and an HMO of 40,000 would need 0.4 FTE psychiatrists.

The relationship between HMO size and psychiatric FTEs becomes clear if we return to HMO X with 50,000 members, 833 of whom will require psychiatric attention over the course of one year. Most of these 833 individuals—about 80 percent—will need only an initial medication evaluation and two to three follow-up visits for monitoring, adjustment, or discontinuance of psychotropic medication. These sessions can be 10 to 15 minutes in length—one hour or less per person per year, or 666 hours per year total. The remaining 20 percent will require from 30 minutes to an hour of medical-psychiatric evaluation time per person per year, or 167 hours per year total. Therefore, the 833 members will consume only about 833 hours of psychiatric time per year. A 0.5 FTE represents 960 hours per year, leaving 127 hours of the psychiatrist's time as reserve clinical potential.

The other 0.5 FTE of the psychiatrist-director's time is more than sufficient to satisfy the administrative needs of HMO X's department of mental health. In fact, this staffing is not only adequate to take care of administrative duties but allows for following and treating members throughout their hospital course as well. Currently, the average staff or group model HMO with 50,000 members would allocate almost two FTE psychiatrists to do what one FTE is clearly capable of doing. This is not cost-effective staffing; 2.5 to 3.0 FTE mid-level providers could be hired with the money spent on the extra psychiatrist.

Up to what enrollment does this relationship between HMO size and psychiatric FTE hold true? Is there a membership figure beyond which it is no longer valid? The upper limit of enrollment size is between 65,000 and 70,000 members. For example, at an enrollment of 70,000 members, 70 percent of the psychiatrist-director's time will be spent in ambulatory clinical duties, leaving 30 percent for managing the department. Demands for this level of work intensity, and higher, can be made upon psychiatric providers, but the physical and emotional strains are considerable.

I would suggest setting the upper limit of enrollment size for which one psychiatrist-director is responsible at 65,000 members. Beyond 65,000 members, additional psychiatrists can be recruited in increments of 0.25 to 0.30 FTEs for every 25,000 new members (0.30 FTEs instead of 0.25 FTEs per 25,000 new members would provide a reserve of psychiatric clinical potential). This recruitment of additional psychiatric personnel should not be delayed until the 25,000 new members have signed up; hiring should take place early in the process of enrollment—few things are more frustrating than "waiting for the cavalry to arrive."

The new psychiatric recruits should be used as medical subspecialists—that is, for doing medical-psychiatric evaluations and writing prescriptions, as outlined previously. Their work assignments should be carefully regulated by the director to avoid any waste of potential.

At the beginning of this section, I alluded to an alternative method by which psychiatrists can be used. If an HMO elects not to have a psychiatrist-director, then psychiatrists need to be employed in the most efficient and cost-effective manner, that is, as medical subspecialists only. Medical-psychiatric evaluations and prescription writing would be their primary tasks unless they are also hospitalizing and treating the plan's inpatient members. They would work under the supervision of the nonphysician departmental director.

This kind of administrative relationship is, however, fraught with potential difficulties caused by interdisciplinary rivalry and perceived threats to professional status. Except for those in the community mental health sector, most psychiatrists are not used to working under the direction of a nonphysician. Therefore, any possible ambiguity about how power is deployed in the department should be dispelled in the preemployment interview; the "rules of the game" must be made clear to the psychiatrist job applicant.

Because these psychiatrists will be used as medical

subspecialists and not as psychotherapists or managers, they can be recruited in increments of 0.25 to 0.30 FTEs for each block of 25,000 enrollees. It is better to recruit on the high side, 0.30 FTE, in order to have some latitude in provider capacity. This means that in the example of HMO X, with 50,000 members, 0.6 FTE psychiatric provider time would be required.

In summary, this section on psychiatric providers demonstrates three things:

1. There are two ways to deploy psychiatric personnel efficiently and cost-effectively in an HMO department of mental health.

2. The HMO national average psychiatrists-to-enrollees ratio of 1:37,780 could more appropriately be set at 1:65,000.

3. The duties of HMO psychiatric providers can be defined in a concise and operational manner.

MID-LEVEL STAFF RATIOS AND MIX

In approaching the issue of mid-level or line provider staff ratios and their mix, it is worthwhile to point out again that the overall ratio of 1:7,000 members suggested previously does not include psychiatrists. Mid-level providers functioning as psychotherapists render the bulk of direct service in the department and should be considered separately.

Several disciplines are available in the selection of mid-level providers: M.S.W.s, M.S.N.s, R.N.s, and Ph.D.s, M.S.s and M.A.s in psychology. There are even formulas to assist in this selection process.[7] However, as I indicated in chapter 4 in the section on degrees, a great deal of debate about what provider type to choose can be eliminated by employing the concept of role equivalency. What are the required tasks, and what attributes are necessary to accomplish these tasks without regard to specific academic degrees?

If the problem of line staff selection is approached from this operational point of view, then it becomes clear that the main task of the mid-level provider is psychotherapy. More than 90 percent of the clinical work done in an HMO department of mental health, regardless of whether it occurs in groups, families, or individuals, is simply general psychotherapy that can be provided by any of the above disciplines. Thinking in terms of role equivalency makes staff selection much easier for managers. For example, one method of selection is to implement a one-third guideline: one-third social workers, one-third psychiatric nurses, and one-third psychologists. This method provides a balance of available skills and avoids any question of unfair discrimination between disciplines.

The current national average group and staff model staffing ratios for psychiatrists, social workers, psychiatric nurses, and psychologists are shown in Table 7-3.

These figures demonstrate a hiring preference for social workers over psychiatric nurses and psychologists (3.8 social workers for every psychiatric nurse and 1.6 social workers for every psychologist). Although not distributed in a one-third balance, these data, when compared to those from earlier studies, give some indication that forces of equalization in hiring are active. It is to be hoped that this tendency will continue, especially in the case of the psychiatric nurse.

Table 7-3
HMO Provider Ratios by Discipline
(National Average, Group and Staff Model)[2]

Psychiatrist	1:37,780
Social worker	1:21,854
Psychiatric nurse	1:82,805
Psychologist	1:35,786
*Other	1:65,116
Total providers	1:7,521

Listed as associate in arts degree holder, mental health counselor, and mental health technician.

There are indications that the psychiatric clinical nurse specialist has been underutilized in the prepaid sector.[11] The potential of this provider is just now being more fully recognized. Psychiatric clinical nurse specialists are highly trained therapists with strong medical backgrounds who have accumulated a great deal of administrative experience. The team concept of providing service is second nature to them, and their work load capacity is remarkable. Their experience in emergency departments, ICUs, CCUs, and other crisis-oriented units leads to a work esprit and a relative imperturbability that are valuable assets to a department.

Although psychotherapy is by far the major task of line staff in terms of time commitment, psychological testing is also important. Here we encounter an exception to role equivalency; psychologists are uniquely suited by their training to administer and interpret psychological tests. Therefore, their schedules must have enough latitude to reflect this function. But how much latitude? Some departments require that a rather elaborate battery of psychological tests be given to each member seeking mental health service. This practice has a marked impact on available provider time and is unnecessary. Testing should be limited to (1) cases that specifically require it (examples: the need to determine I.Q., or the need to present testing results to courts, schools, or disability review boards) and (2) cases in which testing is needed to supplement clinical data in arriving at a treatment plan (for example, questions of organicity versus functional impairment, or need to determine aptitude and interest when career counseling). An HMO of 100,000 members can more than meet its testing requirements with one FTE psychologist.

Chapter 8
PROVIDER PRODUCTIVITY

Two general methods can be used for developing standards of provider productivity. One involves requiring a set number of encounters per unit time, and the other requires a certain percentage of face-to-face clinical time. Both methods are used in the prepaid sector, and both have adherents who argue the advantage of one system over the other. I use provider productivity standards based on the percentage of clinical time rather than encounters per unit time because the latter system can degenerate into something resembling piecework quotas in a factory. For example, in a department in which a requirement of five or six encounters per day is the standard, there is an incentive to schedule five or six half-hour sessions in the morning and "take the rest of the day off." This is obviously not good practice and should be avoided.

A productivity standard of 80 percent clinical time was used in the previous chapter in determining staffing requirements. Some maintain that 80 percent is too high, but the field's statistics do not support the position that this is excessive. The current national average staff clinical and administrative times in percent by discipline for group and staff model HMOs are shown in Table 8-1.

Table 8-1.
Average Distribution of Clinical and Administrative Time[2]

	Percent Clinical	Percent Administrative
Psychiatrist	85	15
Psychologist	86	14
Social worker	91	9
Psychiatric nurse	93	7
Other	83	17
Overall	88	12

If anything, 80 percent clinical time is on the low side when compared to existing averages in the field. One explanation for the rather high overall national average of 88 percent is that this time figure probably includes no-shows and late cancellations, which can amount to as much as 20 percent of scheduled cases in some departments.[5] My suggested 80 percent clinical time is actual face-to-face time; it does not include no-shows or cancellations.

One method of ensuring that no-shows and cancellations do not reduce clinical time below 80 percent is to schedule line providers at 90 percent clinical time and then have the departmental secretary confirm all scheduled appointments 24 hours in advance. This maneuver will reduce no-shows to a minimum and alert the department to cancellations. Regardless of what standard is set, prior confirmation of appointments should be instituted because this technique averts many hours of wasted provider time.

An issue that always arises when provider productivity is considered is "churning," or scheduling members more frequently than is necessary in order to fill up clinical time with nondemanding cases. Churning is actually a sign that either the provider's morale is low or that his or her attitude is not compatible with HMO work. In either case, the situation requires correction if provider morale in general is to remain high. The best way to detect churning is to review kept appointments periodically. If the same name reappears weekly or biweekly for more than 10 visits, then a quick case review with the provider in question is warranted. This review often discloses that the member is not progressing well and that the 10 visits were justified. Occasionally, however, no justification for continued therapy can be presented, and the problem must be discussed. Some providers will defend this type of overutilization by claiming a personal need to do long-term therapy regardless of the member's need. This potential impasse is averted in some HMOs by means of a policy allowing two or three long-term therapy cases for each provider.

I take a hard-nosed stand on this: If the member doesn't require the extra sessions, then the overutilization encourages dependency and is therefore contraindicated. If the provider is adamant about doing long-term therapy, then the fee-for-service sector might be better able to use these talents.

Chapter 9
UTILIZATION RATES

Two utilization figures must be considered in an HMO department of mental health: the number of yearly ambulatory mental health encounters per member and the hospital bed days per 1,000 members per year.

The national average ambulatory rate for group and staff model plans falls between 0.21[2] and 0.30[12] encounters per member per year. The ambulatory rate is a deceptive index, however. For example, in HMO X, with 50,000 members, an ambulatory rate of 0.30 would indicate that the department generated 15,000 encounters during the year (0.30 x 50,000 = 15,000). Is this commendable or not? It all depends on how the 15,000 encounters were generated: 0.30 encounters per member per year for HMO X could mean that 5 percent of the membership (2,500) were seen for six visits or that 1.5 percent of the membership (750) were seen for 20 visits. Obviously, the first scenario is in keeping with the most likely yearly membership need, whereas the latter probably represents artificially skewed utilization and churning. Therefore, the ambulatory encounter rate is useful only if the other variables, of which it is a product, are known. The ambulatory encounter rate is of limited value in evaluating service delivery, and much more emphasis should be placed on indexes of inpatient utilization.

INPATIENT UTILIZATION DATA

Hospital bed days per 1,000 members per year, as the ambulatory encounter rate, is the product of two variables: the hospitalization rate per 1,000 members per year and the average hospital length of stay. But unlike the ambulatory rate, the hospital bed days figure is vitally important to the departmental budget; it is the figure that causes apoplexy among departmental directors when the hospital bills arrive.

The national average mental health hospital bed day figure for group, staff, and IPA model plans is 32.7.[12] This average has remained virtually stable over the past four years (1982-86), but the range of hospital bed days among plans shows a considerable amount of variation (2.24 to 70.0 hospital bed days).[2] This means that the HMO with the highest inpatient utilization is paying 31.25 times as much per 1,000 members per year for inpatient hospitalization as the plan with the lowest rate. If both high and low plans have 50,000 members, the difference in amounts paid per year is more than $1 million.

A range of this magnitude in utilization indicates that some plans must be approaching their tasks in an entirely different manner from other plans. Are there identifiable practice characteristics in departments with lower than average hospital bed days? The most recent national HMO mental health survey identified six variables associated with lower than average inpatient utilization.

In reviewing the administrative, service delivery, and benefit characteristics of group and staff model HMOs that are related to mental health inpatient utilization, the following was demonstrated:

1. Leaner average overall provider ratios were associated with lower hospital bed days.

2. Higher provider clinical times were associated with lower hospital bed days.

3. Weekly departmental staff meetings were associated with lower hospital bed days.

4. Shorter waiting times for routine initial evaluations and follow-up visits were associated with lower hospital bed days.

5. The presence of a mutually agreed-upon model (usually short-term, goal-oriented problem solving) for service delivery was associated with lower hospital bed days.

6. The presence of a limitation on inpatient coverage for noncompliant patients was associated with lower hospital bed days.[2]

Some of the survey's findings require further explanation. Number 1 was the unexpected empirical finding that those plans with below-average hospital bed days had an average overall provider ratio of 1:8,506, whereas those plans with above-average hospital bed days had an average overall provider ratio of 1:5,803. In other words, the more available the providers, the higher the inpatient utilization. The survey's authors attributed this paradox to a shift in focus from utilization goals to a focus on work load in those departments experiencing above-average inpatient utilization. Numbers 3 and 5, the presence of a weekly departmental staff meeting and a mutually agreed-upon model of service delivery, are characteristics of an integrated and well-ordered mental health service and are in perfect harmony with lower than average hospital bed days. The finding in number 6 regarding lower hospital bed days in plans limiting inpatient coverage for noncompliant members is also predictable. As the survey's authors put it, "Since this category of patient not only consumes an inordinate amount of provider time but is also more prone to seek inappropriate inpatient care, it makes sense that those plans with a definite policy for limiting their access to hospital will experience lower inpatient utilization."[2]

Length of Stay vs. Hospitalization Rate

The survey provided useful information regarding current prepaid practice but remained silent about the two variables that make up hospital bed days: average length of stay and hospitalization rate. Unless these factors are known, it is impossible to analyze a department's inpatient utilization performance in any but the most general manner. For example, in HMO X we might see a figure of 30 hospital bed days reported. Thirty is about the national average rate, but that is all that can be determined from this figure alone. It could mean that the average length of stay was five days and the hospitalization rate was 6.0 hospitalizations per 1,000 members per year (300). It could also mean that the average length of stay was 30 days and the hospitalization rate was 1.0 (50). The first scenario would indicate that inpatient stay was approaching the ideal, but that ambulatory service delivery was in chaos. The second set of figures would indicate the converse; that is, ambulatory services were being delivered efficiently, but marked overutilization was occurring on the inpatient side. In the former situation, corrective action would have to occur on the ambulatory side, but in the latter, new arrangements would have to be made in the agreements for hospitalization.

INDIVIDUAL PLAN UTILIZATION DATA

At this point I want to outline and discuss inpatient utilization data of mental health departments with which I have had experience. Table 9-1 reflects inpatient utilization (mental health and substance abuse combined) for the years 1979 through 1983, during which time I directed the department of mental health at Group Health Plan of Southeast Michigan (GHP). Table 9-2 reflects my group's inpatient utilization (mental health only) for the years 1984 through 1986 while under contract with Health Alliance Plan (HAP). The averages from Tables 9-1 and 9-2 cannot be combined because the 1979-1983 data included substance abuse, whereas the 1984-1986 data is for mental health only. It should be kept in mind that the average HMO hospitalization rate is 3.0, that the average length of stay is about 10.9 days, and that the average number of hospital bed days is 32.7.

Table 9-1.
Inpatient Utilization, GHP

Year	Enrollment	Hospital Bed Days per 1,000 Members	Average Length of Stay (in Days)	Hospitalization Rate
1979	12,000	13.80	13.8	1.00
1980	16,000	4.56	14.7	0.31
1981	22,000	6.72	16.8	0.40
1982	26,000	4.82	9.1	0.53
1983	29,000	4.65	7.5	0.62
Average	21,000	6.91	12.4	0.57

Table 9-2.
Inpatient Utilization, HAP

Year	Enrollment	Hospital Bed Days per 1,000 Members	Average Length of Stay (in Days)	Hospitalization Rate
1984	24,500	7.31	11.6	0.63
1985	25,000	5.89	10.9	0.54
1986	27,000	6.25	11.8	0.53
Average	25,500	6.48	11.4	0.57

Despite the fact that data from Tables 9-1 and 9-2 cannot be combined, they demonstrate consistent trends in hospital bed days, average lengths of stay, and hospitalization rates that are compatible with effective HMO practice. The overall hospital bed days are less than 22 percent of the national average for HMOs. This means that my departments generated costs of less than 22 percent of those departments at the national average and less than 10 percent of those departments at the upper range of hospital bed days. How was this done? Examine the hospitalization rates in Tables 9-1 and 9-2. On average, they are less than 20 percent of the national average rate of 3.0. Here's the *sine qua non* of an efficient and cost-contained HMO mental health department—a low hospitalization rate. By the vigorous use of crisis intervention techniques and community mental health concepts, it is possible to reduce the mental health hospitalization rate to a fraction of the national average rate.

A low hospitalization rate implies that members who are hospitalized will manifest significant emotional disturbance and might well require more than the national average length of stay. This was indeed the case with our members; their average length of stay was slightly above the national average of 10.9 days.

These rates were generated with a staff that was not particularly large in comparison to the national HMO average. Our overall providers-to-enrollees ratio at GHP varied between 1:6,000 and 1:8,500; the present ratio at HAP is 1:9,375.

The information in Tables 9-1 and 9-2 should be sufficient to prompt HMO managers who are responsible for cost containment to reevaluate national average inpatient utilization figures for mental health. It is to be hoped that the managers will realize that these "fixed" averages are far in excess of what they should be and that they will actively encourage their own mental health departments to become more efficient and cost effective. Contrary to what some internal critics of prepaid mental health service say, it is not a nickel and dime expenditure. In HMO X, for example, the difference in yearly cost between the national average inpatient utilization and 10 hospital bed days is more than $350,000; for each 10 hospital bed days above the national average, add another $175,000.

It's not that difficult to break the 32.7 "barrier" and achieve hospital bed day levels of 10 to 12. However, doing this requires a department in which the entire staff agrees with and implements HMO-compatible patterns of practice. There is no place for fee-for-service orientation in an efficient and cost-effective HMO department of mental health.

Chapter 10
QUALITY ASSURANCE

It is generally agreed that an internal assessment program is necessary for the effective and accountable operation of an HMO mental health department. Therefore, the question is not one of whether there will or will not be a quality assurance (QA) program, but rather one of who will conduct the program and how.

The director should take a very active role in developing, implementing, and maintaining a QA program in the department. Ultimate responsibility for these tasks should not be delegated to subordinates, nor should these tasks be imposed on personnel outside the department. This does not imply that the director should not assign specific QA tasks or accept input from outside the department; it simply means that QA is such an important function that internal control of it should be maintained.

How an internal assessment program is conducted is governed by a rather rigid requirement: It must satisfy the standards and procedures of an external assessment organization. In some ways, this requirement is unfortunate because it limits innovation, but the overall effect of creating uniform measures of quality probably outweighs any potential loss of inventiveness.

The general standards for external assessment will be the same whether the internal assessment entity addresses issues of structure, process, or outcome. The following summary of these general standards can be used as an outline for developing internal assessment policies and procedures:

1. A defined internal organizational structure for the QA program must be developed. This means that an identified individual or committee must be chosen to conduct the program, with input from the entire staff. Regularly scheduled, documented meetings must be held to address QA issues, and the written records of these meetings must be given to the individual or committee responsible for overall QA in the HMO.

2. Defined and comprehensive procedures for the identification and selection of actual and potential problems must be developed. This means developing written procedures for gathering information about actual and potential mental health problem areas in the department and in

the other services as well (the information input must have a broad base). Written procedures must be developed for selecting and judging the importance of the problem areas.

3. Defined and comprehensive procedures for problem evaluation must be developed. These written procedures must include screening criteria for problem selection, proof of adequate samples to perform an analysis, and an outline of the actual process of analysis.

4. Defined and comprehensive procedures for making and implementing appropriate recommendations must be developed. The recommendations should be feasible and written (even if the recommendation is for no action) and given to an individual(s) formally assigned to implement them.

5. Defined and comprehensive procedures for follow-up on the recommendation must be developed. This involves developing written assessment or reaudit procedures along with procedures for revision and/or continued monitoring of the recommendation process when necessary. Follow-up results must be given in writing to the individual or committee responsible for overall QA in the HMO.

Regardless of the present intensity of external scrutiny, a formal, documented QA program should be made operational in every HMO department of mental health. Setting up such a program not only anticipates more stringent assessment regulation but also serves to clarify and focus departmental attention on problem areas such as overutilization, member dissatisfaction, program inadequacy, and barriers to access. A comprehensive QA program can be expected to heighten quality of service and help in cost containment as well.

One of the arguments against developing an adequate QA program is its cost. Granted, it is costly to develop a set of written procedures that comply with the standards of an external assessment organization, but developing them is a one-time expenditure. Once the QA program is in place, the cost of maintaining it can be nominal.[13] On the other hand, identifying and eliminating one cause of overutilization, be it procedure- or provider-based, can pay for the entire QA program for several years.

The following documents are examples of QA instruments currently being used in the prepaid field. With whatever changes that might be required to make them appropriate for a specific organization, they can function as guidelines for developing QA indexes.

MEMBER SATISFACTION SURVEY

This survey is a useful tool for monitoring the overall satisfaction level of members who are receiving mental health services. On occasion, it can provide valuable information regarding previously undetected problem areas in service delivery.

The time interval at which this survey can be administered is arbitrary; for example, it can be applied to all mental health encounters during a three-day period once every six months, or perhaps to all mental health encounters during a five-day period once a year. The important thing to remember is that it must be applied to *all encounters* during the period of sampling.

Member Satisfaction Survey

Overall care and attention: Excellent _____
Good _____
Not too good _____
Poor _____

	Excellent	Good	Not Too Good	Poor
Mental health appointments people and procedures	___	___	___	___
Care by mental health staff	___	___	___	___
Cleanliness and appearance of health center	___	___	___	___
Problems/complaints about mental health service have been taken care of	___	___	___	___

			Yes	No
Mental health staff are reasonably prompt				
Mental health staff seem interested in you and your health			___	___
Mental health staff give good personal attention			___	___
Mental health staff are courteous			___	___
In your opinion, we give you enough information about your problem			___	___
Do you feel you can recommend the mental health department to friends and others?			___	___

Comments:

MEMBER GRIEVANCE FORM

This form is general in nature and can be used in any department of the HMO to document the member grievance process from initiation to disposition. In most HMOs, this process is initiated in the the office of membership services, although there is some variation in this policy throughout the field.

Member Grievance Form

Member name _____ Complaint received ____ In person

Medical record no._____ ____ In writing

____ By telephone

Person initiating form _____ Date received _____

1. Describe complaint (be specific, i.e., date of incident(s), names, etc.):

Signature _____ Date ____ / ____ / ____

2. Investigation:

Signature _____ Date ____ / ____ / ____

Refer to _____

3. Action taken/disposition:

PROVIDER PRODUCTIVITY FORM

This form can be used periodically to monitor the provider productivity aspect of QA. The instrument measures productivity both in terms of the percentage of time spent in direct face-to-face clinical service per day and the total number of encounters per day. As mentioned in chapter 8 on provider productivity, the author prefers the standard of percentage of clinical time, but many departments measure productivity by total encounters. An obvious advantage of this form is that it yields both measures of provider productivity on one index.

Provider Productivity Form

_____
(Therapist)

_____
(Date)

Time	Service (Individual, Family, Group, Administrative Time, etc.)	No. of Patient Encounters
9:00		
9:30		
10:00		
10:30		
11:00		
11:30		
12:00		
12:30		

Percentage of time spent in direct service: _____ Total encounters: _____

PEER CASE REVIEW

This form can be used to document an essential aspect of a plan's QA program: peer review. The instrument is brief, but it includes the necessary categories for effective peer review.

Peer Case Review

Date: _____

Medical Record No. _____ Source of referral _____

Sex _____ Age _____ Diagnosis _____

Case summary:

Discussion and recommendations:

Therapist_____

Peer review committee

_____

_____

_____

BASIC PRINCIPLES FOR DOCUMENTATION

A guideline of this sort should appear not only in the QA manual but in the department's general policy and procedure manual as well. Making it part of the policy and procedure manual increases the likelihood that the staff will be exposed to it and thereby incorporate these important rules into their record keeping.

1. Make sure that you are writing in the right record. Double-check the patient's name, medical record number, and age. Keep in mind that two or more patients may have the same name (fathers and sons, for example), so it is important that the record be checked.

2. All entries must be neat, legible, and in black ballpoint ink.

3. All entries must be dated.

4. Be complete, using good judgment as a guide when charting. Remember that the record may be seen by the patient, parents or guardian, attorneys, etc.

   (a) Use the SOAP (Subjective Objective Assessment Plan) format whenever possible.

   (b) Document the important information—patient's chief complaint, symptoms, subjective findings, objective findings, diagnosis, instructions to the patient, prescriptions, diagnostic tests, referrals, instructions for follow-up visits. Telephone calls must be documented thoroughly. Be sure to indicate that the contact was a telephone call.

   (c) If a patient refuses treatment, advice, or hospitalization, or states that he or she doesn't want to know the risks or side effects of a treatment, be sure that these statements are documented. Document when a patient fails to comply with prescribed treatment. Document that implications were explained to the patient.

   (d) Avoid criticism of other professionals or departments.

   (e) Do not load the chart with long, defensive, or unnecessary notes.

   (f) The record should reflect the complexity of a difficult clinical problem. If it does, it will demonstrate to a court that proper professional attention has been given to the problem.

The record is the most important element in a malpractice litigation. It reveals what happened, what didn't happen, when, why (or why not), how, who, etc. A rule of thumb often used in malpractice litigation is, "If it is not charted, it did not happen."

5. Use only standard abbreviations and symbols. When the meaning of any abbreviation is not clear to the layman, it might be wise to spell out the abbreviated phrase in full.

6. To correct errors:

   (a) Leave the original record intact with *a single line* drawn through the entry being corrected.

   (b) Write "error" and initials above the entry or in the margins of the line that is in error.

   (c) Do not use correction fluid in the record.

   (d) Do not erase an entry.

   (e) Do not put in arrows to add information. It is best to cross out and rewrite the entry correctly. If information must be added later, or if an error is noted at a later time, be sure to note the date and time of the addition or correction. *It is always better for the record to show an error in record-keeping than for the recorder to be suspected of tampering with or falsifying a record.*

7. Do not skip lines or leave blanks in the record. Draw a line through any empty space at the end of an entry to the end of the page.

8. All entries must be signed. It is preferable to use full name and title, but the entries may be signed with the provider's signature as documented in the signature book. All physicians' orders must be cosigned by the nurse or medical assistant carrying out those orders. Initials may be used to cosign.

9. Records must be completed promptly while the staff's memories are fresh.

10. All consultant reports, emergency department reports, hospital records, previous physicians' records, and diagnostic test reports must be reviewed and initialed by a provider.

11. The patient's name and medical record number must appear on every page of the medical record.

12. Medical records may not be taken from the clinic except to be transferred from one center to another.

13. Confidentiality must be maintained at all times.

A good medical record is carefully prepared, complete, accurate, legible, relevant, timely, and generously informative.

MEASUREMENT OF OUTCOME

The following two documents are questionnaires that attempt to measure the nebulous but all-important aspect of QA known as outcome. The first instrument, Confidential Personal Progress Questionnaire, was designed for use with adult members seeking mental health service for themselves. The second instrument, Confidential Parent Questionnaire, was designed for use with the parents (or guardians) of children receiving mental health service.

The appropriate questionnaire can be given to randomly selected members, with follow-up after a predetermined interval—for example, after three months or six months of therapy. To ensure comparability, the follow-up questionnaires are identical to the forms shown here, with the exception that the instructional statement at the beginning of each form is revised.

Confidential Personal Progress Questionnaire

Name_____ Date _____ Medical Record No. _____

So that you and your therapist may better understand your situation, and so that we may be able to see your progress in therapy, we are asking that you take a few minutes to answer the following questions. We will ask these questions when you begin treatment and again when therapy nears completion. This will give both you and your therapist a chance to judge how much you have improved as a result of coming to our department. We encourage you to talk over your ideas about treatment with your therapist; your ideas, expectations, fears, and needs are very important.

We are also interested in getting your opinion of the care you receive here and will ask you to tell us how satisfied you were with our services near the completion of your therapy.

Regarding Your Problems

Please note the extent to which the following have been a problem in the past seven days (including today).

None means "has not occurred at all."
Mild means "has occurred but has not gotten in the way of my usual activities."
Moderate means "has occurred and gotten in the way of some of my usual activities."
Severe means "has occurred frequently and has kept me from doing a lot of things or made me do things I didn't want to do."

Your thinking:	None/Not A Problem	A Mild Problem	Moderate Problem	Severe Problem
1. Trouble concentrating	___	___	___	___
2. Having upsetting thoughts ...	___	___	___	___

3. Feeling self-conscious .... ___   ___   ___   ___
4. Trouble controlling thoughts .. ___   ___   ___   ___

Your feelings:

5. Feel tense, anxious, or nervous ___   ___   ___   ___
6. Feel sad or depressed .... ___   ___   ___   ___
7. Feel fearful or afraid .... ___   ___   ___   ___
8. Feel angry or irritable .... ___   ___   ___   ___

Your physical health:

9. Have too much energy .... ___   ___   ___   ___
10. Have too little energy .... ___   ___   ___   ___
11. Have physical problems
(headaches, backaches, etc.) ... ___   ___   ___   ___
12. Sleep too much .... ___   ___   ___   ___
13. Have trouble falling asleep or
staying asleep .... ___   ___   ___   ___
14. Eat too much .... ___   ___   ___   ___
15. Have no appetite .... ___   ___   ___   ___

Your behavior:

16. Have acted nervous or jittery .. ___   ___   ___   ___
17. Have had unwanted or
irritating habits .... ___   ___   ___   ___
18. Have had difficulty with alcohol ___   ___   ___   ___
19. Have had difficulty with pills or
drugs .... ___   ___   ___   ___
20. Have had difficulty in using
spare time well .... ___   ___   ___   ___

Getting along with others:

21. Have avoided being around
people .... ___   ___   ___   ___
22. Have had disagreements with
people .... ___   ___   ___   ___
23. Believe others have rejected me ___   ___   ___   ___
24. Believe others have pressured
me to do things .... ___   ___   ___   ___
25. Have spent most of my time
alone .... ___   ___   ___   ___
26. Have had trouble saying what
was on my mind .... ___   ___   ___   ___

List any other problems you would like to deal with in therapy:

Thank you for your cooperation.

Confidential Parent Questionnaire

Name_____ Date _____ Medical Record No. _____

So that you and your child's therapist may better understand your child's situation, and so that we may be able to see your child's progress after therapy is completed, we are asking that you take a few minutes to answer the following questions. We will ask these questions when your child begins treatment and again when therapy is ended. This will give both you and your child's therapist a chance to judge how much your child has improved as a result of coming to our department. We encourage you to talk over your ideas about treatment with your child's therapist—your ideas, expectations, fears, and needs are very important.

We are also interested in getting your opinion of the care your child receives here and will ask you to tell us how satisfied you were with our services near the completion of your child's therapy.

Please note the extent to which the following have been a problem for your child in the past *month*. Please answer all questions. Beside each item please indicate the seriousness of the of the problem by a check mark under the proper response.

	Not At All	Just a Little	Pretty Much	Very Much
Your child's learning/motivation:				
1. Has difficulty in learning	—	—	—	—
2. Fails to finish tasks	—	—	—	—
3. Is childish or immature (wants help he or she shouldn't need, needs constant reassurance)	—	—	—	—
4. Is easily frustrated in doing tasks	—	—	—	—
5. Has an "I don't care" attitude	—	—	—	—
Your child's activity level:				
6. Is excitable, impulsive	—	—	—	—
7. Is restless (unable to sit still)	—	—	—	—
8. Is restless (up and on the go)	—	—	—	—
9. Distractibility or attention span is a problem	—	—	—	—
10. Mood changes quickly and drastically	—	—	—	—
Your child's anxiety/withdrawal:				
11. Sucks or chews (thumb, clothing, blanket)	—	—	—	—
12. Cries easily	—	—	—	—

13. Is fearful (of new situations, new
    people or places, going to school, etc.) ____ ____ ____ ____
14. Acts shy . . . . ____ ____ ____ ____
15. Worries more than others (about being
    alone, illness, death, etc.) . . . . ____ ____ ____ ____
16. Withdraws quickly from group
    activities, prefers to be alone . . . . ____ ____ ____ ____

Your child's conduct with adults/rules:

17. Is sassy to grown-ups . . . . ____ ____ ____ ____
18. Carries a chip on shoulder . . . . ____ ____ ____ ____
19. Is destructive . . . . ____ ____ ____ ____
20. Denies mistakes or blames others . . . . ____ ____ ____ ____
21. Is quarrelsome, argumentative . . . . . . ____ ____ ____ ____
22. Steals . . . . ____ ____ ____ ____
23. Is disobedient or obeys resentfully . . . ____ ____ ____ ____

Your child's relations with other children:

24. Bullies others . . . . ____ ____ ____ ____
25. Fights . . . . ____ ____ ____ ____
26. Has problems with making or keeping
    friends . . . . ____ ____ ____ ____
27. Has difficulty in getting along with
    brothers or sisters . . . . ____ ____ ____ ____

Your child's physical health:

28. Has headaches . . . . ____ ____ ____ ____
29. Has problems with eating (poor
    appetite, leaves table between bites) . . ____ ____ ____ ____
30. Complains of stomach-aches . . . . ____ ____ ____ ____
31. Has problems with sleep (can't fall
    asleep, tosses and turns, up in the
    night, etc.) . . . . ____ ____ ____ ____
32. Complains of other aches and pains . . ____ ____ ____ ____
33. Has vomiting or nausea . . . . ____ ____ ____ ____
34. Wets bed or clothing . . . . ____ ____ ____ ____
35. Goes to bathroom too frequently . . . . ____ ____ ____ ____
36. Soils clothing . . . . ____ ____ ____ ____

Your child's thinking and feeling:

37. Is depressed, unhappy, sad . . . . ____ ____ ____ ____
38. Has problems expressing emotions . . ____ ____ ____ ____

39. Shows excessive fantasy (imaginary persons, monsters, etc.) . . . .   ___   ___   ___   ___
40. Shows weird or bizarre behavior . . . . .   ___   ___   ___   ___
41. Seems unaware of what is going on . . .   ___   ___   ___   ___

List any other problems you would like to deal with in therapy:

Thank you for your cooperation.

Chapter 11
POLICIES AND PROCEDURES

For most clinicians, paperwork is a bane that they will do almost anything to avoid. This is understandable, since therapy is more art than science. "Leave policy and procedure development to the administrators—I can't be bothered," cries the therapist. Although one can sympathize with this statement on a feeling level, it must be rejected on a rational level. If clinicians don't write their own rules of practice, nonclinicians will do it for them. They are part of a regulated field of endeavor that is becoming more regulated, so it is appropriate that they take an active part in creating the policies and procedures that will govern their professional lives now and in the future.

As in developing a QA program, the positive side of this situation is that once a policy and procedure manual has been written, very few additions to it will be required. Creating a comprehensive document is the initial one-time investment in terms of staff commitment. A major benefit in having a complete policy and procedure manual is cost containment; this is often overlooked, but it is nevertheless a real benefit. For example, the manual can provide standardization and integration of service delivery from center to center within the HMO, guidelines for training new therapists, and protection in malpractice suits by serving as a source for justification of actions.

ISSUES TO BE COVERED

Policy and procedure manuals need not be elaborate, but they should represent what is actually done in the department; written procedures should reflect practice. In some departments, there is little connection between what is written and what is done. The manual is usually far more complicated than the operations it represents. An initial brief outline of the department's general treatment philosophy and goals should be followed by sections containing *short* policy statements and *clear* procedural steps that address key administrative, service delivery, and benefit issues. A partial list of these issues includes:

1. *Intake and triage.* This section should list the steps involved in accepting a referral, includ-

ing examples of intake forms; criteria for evaluating degree of urgency; departmental access standards; and procedures for triage and appropriate follow-up or referral.

2. *Treatment category assignment.* This section should operationalize the clinical decision-making processes that lead to assigning a member to a particular in-house treatment modality (individual, group, couple, family), hospital, another provider outside of the HMO, or determining that no treatment is required.

3. *Hospitalization.* This section deals with *who* is hospitalized (criteria for hospitalization, including benefit interpretations for limitations and exclusions); *where* they are hospitalized (list of approved inpatient facilities along with names and telephone numbers of contact persons); and *how* they are hospitalized (steps for arranging hospitalization, along with copies of all necessary authorization forms). Procedures for monitoring the member's progress, length of stay, and reentrance into the ambulatory system after discharge also should be included in this section.

4. *Medication guidelines.* This section should outline the clinical criteria used to recommend psychotropic medication. It should include a checklist of contraindications to prescribing medication and a protocol for monitoring response, side effects, and need for dosage adjustment, change, or discontinuation of medication. A written copy of instructions to

members regarding the purpose, expected response, possible side effects, and need for compliance with a medication regimen also should be included in this section.

5. *Assessment and management of violent or potentially violent members.* The Tarasoff decision has made it essential that the department not only have documented procedures for the management of violent members but also standards regarding foreseeable violence, potential victim(s), and attempts to protect the potential victim(s). This last standard involves written or verbal warnings, which must be documented. This section is extremely important because there is evidence that recent court decisions represent a trend to impose strict liability on providers for any violent acts committed by those under their care.[14]

6. *Guidelines for determining and reporting actual and suspected child abuse.* As in the Tarasoff decision, the law of negligence applies here. Therefore, written criteria for evaluating and reporting child abuse must be developed. Child protective service agencies often provide copies of the statutes governing this problem area; these can be included in this section.

7. *Obtaining legal advice.* Providers sometimes find themselves in emergency situations that have potential adverse legal consequences. Therefore, the name, phone number, and procedure for contacting the plan's legal counsel

should be drawn up and made part of this section.

8. *Release of information.* This section should include copies of the HMO's release of information forms, statements regarding the purpose of obtaining information, a copy of any instructions given to members on this issue, and a set of *very clear* steps to verify the authenticity and appropriateness of any request for information received from other individuals or organizations. This last process is usually handled by the medical record department, but the mental health department should have final control over what information is released from its case records.

9. *Member grievances.* This section should list all the steps by which a grievance is processed, from initiation to final disposition. A copy of the member grievance form containing space for member identification data, description of the complaint, investigation, and disposition should be included in this section.

10. *No-shows and noncompliance.* HMOs having policies and procedures regarding these issues usually incorporate negative sanctions within them. The sanctions can range in severity from charging for a missed appointment to limitation or outright exclusion of service. Because the topics of service limitation and exclusion will be considered later in this chapter, it is sufficient at this point to suggest that any policy or procedure in this area be carefully documented.

11. *Use of community resources.* This section contains guidelines for use of a community resource handbook (either the official county edition or a listing compiled by the department). The guidelines should list criteria used in making a referral (wife-battering, child abuse, bankruptcy, legal assistance, etc.), what information should or should not be released to the community resource, and steps for follow-up of the member after referral.

12. *Consultation and education (C & E).* Although C & E is more often associated with community mental health centers (CMHCs) than with HMOs, these are useful and legitimate functions of the HMO department of mental health that should be reflected in the policy and procedure manual. C & E directed to outside agencies and organizations for the purpose of public relations and marketing was discussed in chapter 3. These functions should also be directed internally in the form of in-service training sessions for providers in other services and for select managerial personnel. C & E of this sort can improve service delivery and reduce costs by educating nonmental health providers in techniques of early detection and referral (or treatment) of high-risk members. Managerial personnel also can keep posted on current issues in the mental health department by means of these sessions. The policy and procedure statements in this section should include the goals of C & E and the operational steps used to implement both the external and internal parts of the program.

13. *Outreach programs.* As with C & E, outreach is frequently associated with CMHCs, but this function can be used to good advantage in HMOs as well. Conflict over turf occasionally arises here between those who feel that a health education department should develop and implement mental health outreach and those who feel the task is more properly assigned to the mental health department. A resolution to this kind of strife may be in the recognition that, regardless of who nominally controls the outreach program, the mental health input must come from the mental health department; no other group in the HMO has the required expertise. Therefore, the department's policy and procedure manual should contain a description of the process used to identify problems suitable for outreach (alcoholism, child abuse, chronic overspending, etc.), and an outline of the operations and personnel used to correct these problems (a monthly lecture by the departmental provider with the greatest knowledge in a particular area, a film series on stress management, relaxation techniques, etc., or informational articles included in the regular mailing to enrollees or made available as a handout in the clinic).

14. *Personnel decisions.* This section should include criteria for hiring and evaluation and steps to implement promotions and disciplinary actions. Copies of personnel forms also should be part of this section. The final wording of these criteria and operational steps

should be formulated with the assistance of the HMO's personnel department. Close collaboration with the personnel department is very important because expertise in labor law is required in drafting this section.

As indicated above, this is only a partial list of matters that should be included in a policy and procedure manual. Any administrative, service delivery, or benefit issue that is distinct or has legal or medicolegal implications should be addressed in a separate section.

The issues of benefit limitation and benefit exclusion are policy matters of particular importance to an HMO department of mental health. Most plans have a general policy limitation on mental health benefits: Service is limited to conditions that are not chronic and are likely to respond to short-term therapy. But a general statement of this sort raises several questions. What limitations? What is meant by chronic? What constitutes short-term therapy? Therefore, benefit interpretations in this area must be operationalized in order to have any meaning and to avoid medicolegal controversy.

In an article published in 1985, Bonstedt and McSweeny were the first to comprehensively address the issue of psychiatric limitations and exclusions in HMOs.[15] Following is a synthesis of concepts in their paper, current data from the 1986 national HMO mental health survey referred to previously, and my own experience.

The rationale for the existence of a limitation and exclusion policy is cost containment. HMO actuaries are still haunted by the specter of the bottomless pit phenomenon when it comes to mental health benefits. They are all too aware of the disasters Blue Cross/Blue

Shield suffered in the 1970s after increasing covered mental health benefits for the automotive workers and other employee groups.[16] As a result of the concern about runaway costs, most HMOs limit services to categories of members that are expected to demonstrate disproportionately high utilization. Table 11-1 shows the percentage of group and staff model HMOs which have inpatient limitations on various categories of members.

Table 11-1.
Percent of Group and Staff Plans with Limitations on Inpatient Coverage[2]

Member Category	Percent of Plans with Limitations
Chronic alcoholics	86.8
Chronic drug abusers	90.6
Chronic mentally ill	92.3
Mentally retarded	79.0
Noncompliant	76.6

Comparable figures were obtained for independent practice association models in this national survey, but the number of plans responding was not large enough to produce statistically reliable data.[2]

The data in Table 11-1, combined with inpatient utilization figures from the same study, support the belief that limitations are necessary if costs are to be controlled. Only 66.7 percent of plans with hospital bed days over the national average had a limitation on inpatient coverage for noncompliant members, whereas 85.6 percent of plans with hospital bed days below the national average had some form of inpatient benefit limitation on this group of enrollees.[2] Because this membership category not only consumes an inordinate amount of provider time but is more prone to seek inappropriate inpatient care, it makes sense that those plans with a definite policy for limiting their access to a hospital will experience lower inpatient utilization.

Arriving at a general consensus that limitations and even exclusions are necessary is not a problem. The real issue is how to frame these negative sanctions in policies and procedures so that they are (1) clear and not open to misunderstanding, (2) clinically valid, (3) equitable to the entire membership, and (4) defensible in court. These requirements may appear to be straightforward, but they are fraught with pitfalls for the unwary.

For example, the use of diagnosis as a criterion of chronicity and prognosis would seem to be reasonable. Certain diagnoses would imply conditions that are chronic and not subject to improvement by the use of short-term therapy. By using these standards, service limitations and exclusions could be applied to the diagnostic categories of personality disorders and chronic psychoses. These standards may be reasonable, but they are absolutely useless in drawing up policies and procedures for mental health benefits. The problem here is the notorious unreliability of diagnosis in mental health. If we were dealing with concern about the diagnosis of an astrocytoma versus a meningioma there would be little controversy—but mental health care is not neurosurgery. Every day our courts witness the spectacle of psychiatrists for the prosecution maintaining that a defendant is characterologically impaired and therefore responsible, and psychiatrists for the defense maintaining that this same defendant is psychotic and therefore not responsible. Scenes like this go a long way toward creating and maintaining a negative stereotype of the psychiatrist as either fool or knave. The problem is compounded by the acceptance of multiple diagnoses: The member that is excluded from inpatient service with the diagnosis of chronic antisocial personality disorder may defend himself at his trial for aggravated assault and attack the physician at his trial for malpractice with the diagnosis of acute anxiety disorder.

If diagnosis is open to misunderstanding and not defensible in court, what criteria of chronicity and prognosis can be used? The three most objective and most commonly used standards involve (1) the number of previous psychiatric hospitalizations the member has experienced, (2) the member's degree of disability, and (3) the member's degree of cooperation with a treatment plan.

Using the number of previous psychiatric hospitalizations as a standard requires setting an arbitrary number of previous hospitalizations (in most plans 3 or 4), carefully defining which services are limited or excluded after this number has been reached (in most plans, mental health inpatient coverage is excluded), and listing what documentation is required in order to place a member in this category (usually hospital records or the member's statement, not statements from relatives or friends). All this must be clearly stated in the policy and procedure manual along with steps which the member can take to appeal the decision.

A member's degree of disability is less arbitrary than the previous standard. Here chronicity is defined in terms of the member's eligibility to receive mental health disability benefits. The process requires that the determination be made by an outside agency such as the Social Security Administration or the Veterans Administration, and not the HMO. Once this determination of chronicity has been made, most plans will exclude mental health inpatient service. The relevant phraseology in the benefit interpretation is usually ". . . receiving federal social security disability benefits because of a psychiatric condition" or "The member is an adult dependent, per Internal Revenue Service definition, because of a psychiatric condition." As with the previous standard, all this must be clearly outlined in the policy and procedure manual along with steps by which the member can appeal the decision.

The member's degree of cooperation with a treatment plan is probably the most arbitrary of all standards used to limit or exclude service. Therefore, rules for careful documentation of the initial evaluation, case formulation, treatment plan, and instructions to the member must be developed and made part of the manual. Steps for gathering evidence that the member failed to cooperate (missed appointments, failure to comply with medication regimen, threatening behavior, etc.), along with steps for alerting the member to his or her potential loss of benefits (registered letter, phone calls, face-to-face communication), must also be covered by policy and procedure statements. The entire standard must be operationalized in the policy and procedure manual along with rules governing the appeal process.

In implementing these standards, most plans elect the policy of exclusion. They exclude any mental health inpatient coverage for members who meet any of the above criteria for chronicity or poor prognosis. Excluding inpatient coverage while maintaining ambulatory benefits is probably the best course of action here, inasmuch as this policy allows continuity of service while fostering an incentive in the member to comply with treatment recommendations.

It should be kept in mind that the entire issue of benefit limitations and exclusions is controversial and may well be a subject of future litigation. If this happens, then present standards may have to be revised or discarded. There seems to be a growing concern in the prepaid mental health care sector about allegations of cost shifting to the public sector secondary to the use of limitation and exclusion policies. Debate about the validity of these allegations is beyond the scope of this book, but HMO managers and mental health departmental directors should be aware that the issue is far from settled.

In summary, some forms of safeguard against runaway costs due to chronicity or lack of cooperation are obviously necessary for conducting an efficient and cost-contained HMO department of mental health. The standards used in these safeguards must be operationalized and carefully documented, however. This is not an area in which it is wise to trust to chance.

Chapter 12
INPATIENT PROVIDERS

U p to this point, the emphasis in this book has been on developing and maintaining a high-quality ambulatory structure of service delivery that avoids unnecessary hospitalizations. A low hospitalization rate is the key to a low hospital bed day figure, and ambulatory service is the make-or-break element there. However, no matter what level of efficiency is reached in ambulatory service, there will still be inpatient admissions. How, then, can the average length of stay (ALOS) be kept to a minimum? What can be done to avoid a phenomenon known as the "disappearing member syndrome"—inordinately long inpatient stays due to the HMO's apparent inability to institute effective monitoring procedures while the member is in the hospital? This is a real and costly problem for many HMOs, inasmuch as most plans do not own hospitals.

I used the qualifying adjective above because an HMO's inability to come to a satisfactory agreement with the service area's inpatient providers on ALOS is often more apparent than real. It is a matter of remaining firm with providers and pointing out the reality of recent changes in enrollment statistics and the benefits of cooperating with the plan in achieving a reasonable ALOS for its members. This is not an easy task, but it can be done.

EVALUATING LENGTH OF STAY

First of all, evaluate the present overall ALOS. If it is eight days or less, and the hospitalization rate is acceptable (that is, ±1.0 hospitalizations per 1,000 members per year), this is probably the best figure that can be expected. If the ALOS is more than 12 days, then admission data should be analyzed for the purpose of identifying inpatient providers who are generating ALOS of 10 days or less. This kind of project requires some extra time, but it will more than pay for itself if even one or two outside providers can be found who are not overutilizing the plan's inpatient benefit. If psychiatrists of this sort can be identified, then serious consideration should be given to establishing a more exclusive agreement with them regarding the plan's inpatient needs. They probably would be more than willing to agree on a 10-day ALOS for the plan's members in exchange for the status of a preferred provider. It should be made clear to them that their preferred provider status depends upon their maintaining a low ALOS and cooperating with other inpatient utilization control efforts of the plan. These additional utilization control efforts include obtaining concurrent clinical data regarding the member's presentation, diagnosis, treatment plan, progress, and expected date of discharge. These kinds of data preferably should be obtained on-site in the hospital by the plan's or the department's utilization coordinator, but that kind of advantageous arrangement may be impossible because of hospital bylaws or resistance from the hospital's administrator.

If a core of providers who are currently rendering acceptable inpatient services to the plan cannot be located, then a search for other providers in the community should be undertaken. This process not only involves an expenditure of time but tedious negotiations as well; again, the time and effort spent here will more than pay for themselves if a workable agreement regarding inpatient utilization can be reached.

Some well-established providers will have no interest in an offer of a preferred provider status. However, a thorough search should turn up at least a few local psychiatrists who can appreciate the advisability of becoming part of the prepaid movement in this early, rapid growth phase of the field. Indeed, one of the most persuasive negotiating stances is the fact that prepaid health care is growing at a rate of 25 percent per year and already has a total enrollment of more than 23.6 million members.

Exploring the CMHCs

Another avenue of search for psychiatrists who would be willing to render an acceptable ALOS in the hospital are the CMHCs. These agencies are becoming aware of the advantages of providing mental health care for HMOs, and in many instances are already actively seeking service agreements. Their experience, expertise, and general philosophy of cost-effective service makes them prime candidates for the provision of inpatient mental health care. Also, a CMHC's comprehensive 24-hour crisis intervention system can be used to avoid unnecessary hospitalizations or to expedite appropriate hospitalization by arranging for their staff to do face-to-face evaluations of members who present during the time when the HMO clinic is closed. This sort of night, weekend, and holiday coverage can be very effective in reducing the plan's hospitalization rate. Actually, any number of arrangements with a CMHC regarding inpatient service are possible without abdicating departmental control over service delivery.

Occasionally, a manager will hesitate to change inpatient providers because of a discounted room rate from the hospital out of which the present providers work. Granted, the discount may amount to $50 a day or so; but an ALOS of 15 days with a discount should be compared to 10 days without a discount. The money saved in discounts is more than offset by the extra five days in an inpatient unit. Therefore, striking a good per diem rate is not necessarily cost effective if the ALOS is too long. All of this can be easily determined by calculating the present ALOS and then doing a little simple projective arithmetic. The major aim, assuming that the inpatient service is of high quality, is to obtain the lowest possible overall ALOS.

Short of an HMO's owning its own hospital, the best arrangement to control inpatient stays is for the HMO's own staff to admit, treat, and discharge members from a local inpatient unit. However, this involves staff privileges for the HMO's mental health provider staff. As anyone in the prepaid sector knows, staff privileges are sometimes difficult or even impossible for HMO providers to obtain. There is no easy solution to this dilemma at present. The level of discrimination varies considerably from hospital to hospital around the country, but it is my impression that restrictions are becoming less severe. One approach to this problem area is to contract for one or two beds, with associated staff privileges, in a local psychiatric inpatient unit. The number of beds contracted should, of course, always be less than the plan's expected daily occupancy rate; otherwise, a waste factor would be built in and the plan would be paying for empty beds. The financial arrangement could be on a fixed-fee basis, or could consist of a partial fee plus an extra per diem fee for every day of occupancy. Arrangements of this sort are becoming more likely in the face of the decreased occupancy rates that many hospitals are experiencing. Hospitals, like CMHCs, are starting to reevaluate their stance in relation to the prepaid sector.

Chapter 13
SUBSTANCE ABUSE SERVICE

Although the primary focus of this book has been on the development and delivery of mental health service, some attention should also be given to the issue of substance abuse service in the HMO. This is an important area of health care delivery in any plan and is permeated with misconceptions and controversy.

THE QUESTION OF INTEGRATION

One of the most important questions facing those who are responsible for mental health and substance abuse service development is whether to integrate the two services. Should they be combined into one department or should they be developed independently? No national figures are available on how plans across the country have elected to resolve this question, but it is known that both methods are widely employed. Indeed, a very worthwhile study would be to determine how prepaid plans are actually handling this issue of service integration, and then to do quality and cost analyses of the two administrative options. My prediction is that plans that have combined mental health and substance abuse service delivery would demonstrate higher quality and lower costs than plans in which these services are separate. It should be noted that this outcome prediction is based on experience rather than speculation.

Having developed two HMO departments of mental health over the past nine years, one of them combining mental health and substance abuse and the other keeping the services separate, I have considerable "hands-on" experience as to the pros and cons of both alternatives. In this case, empirical knowledge fits very well into theoretical expectation: Higher quality, greater efficiency, and lower costs are to be expected if similar services are integrated in a unified department.

The major advantage of a unified department is the avoidance of fragmentation of service delivery. On paper, it is quite simple to emphasize the separate and distinct nature of mental health and substance abuse problems, but in practice these distinctions rapidly break down and have no heuristic value. Indeed, if these distinctions are carried to their logical but impractical ends, one encounters the not-that-uncommon scenario of Mr. Jones, who drinks almost a fifth of whiskey a day and is depressed but is unable to receive service in the mental health department because he's an alcoholic and is also unable to receive service in the substance abuse department because he manifests a clinically significant depression. In the course of this avoidance process, the member who requires service simply falls through the cracks in the system and is forgotten until he resurfaces in an out-of-plan substance abuse or mental health unit, or worse. Things like this don't happen if one department has the mandate to treat both mental health and substance abuse problems (assuming, of course, that it is an efficient, well-functioning department).

The concept of a unified department is certainly in agreement with the goals of comprehensiveness and continuity of care. An integrated department can provide the distressed member with a single entry point to a system whose responsibility is to provide holistic treatment and follow-up care for both mental health and substance abuse problems. Departmental policies and procedures should be framed to avoid the kind of fragmentation cited above, which leads to poor quality and cost-ineffective service delivery. Regardless of the magnitude of goodwill and high ethical standards that might exist in separate departments of mental health and substance abuse, jurisdictional and procedural disputes will invariably arise, and invariably the member will suffer, along with the entire system. How much simpler and more efficient it is to combine both types of health care under one aegis and call it the department of mental health.

A method of determining the number of additional providers that would be required if mental health and substance abuse are combined into one department was discussed in chapter 7. Table 7-2 shows that the extra staff requirement in an integrated department is not that large, especially when compared to the advantage gained in efficiency by such an administrative maneuver. For example, in an HMO with 50,000 members, only two full-time equivalent (FTE) additional providers would be required if the services were combined. If substance abuse were a separate department in an HMO of this size, then its number of providers would be between four and five FTEs.

DETERMINING ACCEPTABLE UTILIZATION

The problem of determining acceptable inpatient utilization rates in substance abuse service delivery is more difficult than in mental health because no national average utilization figures are available for the prepaid sector. Substance abuse hospital bed-day figures for individual plans range from less than 1.0 to over 50.0 hospital bed days per 1,000 members per year. As in mental health, variability also seems to be a common theme in substance abuse work.

Societal forces as much as demographics probably influence this utilization rate more than they influence a plan's mental health inpatient utilization rate. The public in general and employers in particular have become increasingly aware of the costly and harmful effects of substance abuse in the United States. The rapid emergence over the past five years of employee assistance programs (EAPs) and union-sponsored educational programs attests to a growing desire to reduce the morbidity and mortality associated with substance abuse. Unfortunately, this concern is often translated into rigid prescriptions to rectify the problem—for example, insisting that the *only* appropriate treatment plan for a substance abuser is a 21- or 28-day intensive inpatient detoxification and treatment program. Plans experience considerable pressure from EAPs, unions, and employers to hospitalize substance abusers regardless of the absence of clinical indications for hospitalization and existing research data demonstrating the advantages of alternative methods of treatment.[17,18] "Considerable pressure" is actually an understatement; "blistering demands" better describes what HMO providers frequently experience while trying to objectively evaluate a case and arrive at the best treatment plan.

Given this milieu, charged with emotion and unrealistic expectations, it is understandable that plans succumb to outside pressure for an across-the-board policy of inpatient hospitalization for substance abusers. Having been on the firing line in this controversy, I can appreciate the temptation to avoid any chance of heated verbal conflict by adopting a stance of acquiescence. This temptation should be resisted, however, because in the last analysis, bad medicine remains bad medicine.

On the brighter side of this issue, educational efforts by HMO providers, although they require considerable time, do have a positive effect in channeling legitimate concern into more appropriate expectations.

Taking the time to outline both the short- and the long-term benefits of a more selective and conservative approach to the treatment of substance abuse is often rewarded by a less dogmatic stance on the part of EAP and union representatives. These educational efforts entail long meetings, conflict, and compromise, but they can result in mutually agreed-upon policies and procedures for the care of substance abusing members.

In conclusion, returning to the problem of determining acceptable inpatient utilization rates for substance abuse, we still face the fact that there are no national average figures for the prepaid sector with which even to begin an analysis. That leaves us with only experience to go on; in most instances, this is the best guide. By referring back to Table 9-1 in chapter 9, it can be seen that my group's *combined* mental health and substance abuse hospital bed days from 1979 through 1983 averaged only 6.91. Unfortunately, we did not construct our data base to differentiate between mental health and substance abuse admissions, but in all likelihood the figure for substance abuse did not exceed 2.0 hospital bed days per 1,000 members per year. Therefore, I would suggest that the following criteria be used in evaluating substance abuse inpatient utilization rates: If the hospital bed days fall between 1 and 5, consider that as acceptable; if they fall between 5 and 10, then some reevaluation of the plan's present mode of service delivery is in order. If hospital bed days are more than 10, then a concerted effort should be made to revamp the substance abuse service delivery system.

Chapter 14
LOOKING AHEAD

As noted before in this volume, the prepaid sector of health care delivery is in the midst of a period of rapid growth, a period that is likely to continue until this mode of health care emerges as the dominant one in this country. An equally dramatic transformation is likely to occur in the manner in which mental health care is delivered; forces already in motion point to the day when short-term therapy, frequently in group form, will supplant long-term, one-on-one therapy, which has been the tradition of the past. Eventually, the concept of peer self-help, already in place in such groups as Alcoholics Anonymous, may actually set aside the need for professional mental health practitioners.

In planning the contents of this book, it was the intention of the author to give major emphasis to those operational elements of an HMO mental health department considered most important in the continued evolution of this mode of health care. But there are other aspects that, even though they might not merit being the focus of an entire chapter, are nonetheless important to the continued progress of HMO-based mental health care as it heads toward the twenty-first century. The five topics covered in this chapter relate more to the "could be" than "what is"; another way of looking at them would be in terms of potential need: Could these activities be of benefit to the organization, the provider, or the prepaid sector as a whole?

DATA COLLECTION, RESEARCH, AND COMMUNICATION

All HMO departments of mental health collect data, but few do research. This situation is not surprising, because the average age of most departments is only eight years.[2] Also, the orientation and priorities of most plans dictate that the major emphasis be placed on service delivery, utilization control, and maintaining a competitive market position. This emphasis does not foster an atmosphere conducive to doing research.

However, the practical need of the HMO to maintain viability is not necessarily in conflict with conducting and publishing research in selected areas. For example, our group went through an extensive trial-

and-error process before we determined the optimum number of sessions for a time-limited couples group of four to five couples. The figure turned out to be nine, with the additional observation that in most cases it could be predicted by the sixth session which couples would benefit from the group. In other words, we developed behavioral criteria that predicted accurately whether a particular couple would or would not experience a significant improvement in their relationship and whether or not the improvement would be maintained for one year.

These were not earth-shattering findings, but they did have practical implications for staffing, scheduling, and ambulatory care costs. Very little extra time would have been required to collect enough data to support a paper on the experience. Publishing is not really a problem at present in HMO work because so little is being written in comparison to the level of reader interest. Unfortunately, our group's orientation at that time was extremely practical, with no interest in research, so a golden opportunity was missed.

About six months after we were sure of our findings, I attended an HMO mental health conference only to find another departmental director informally discussing an identical type of study with identical results. What a waste! The irony here was that neither department considered publishing its results, which had practical value, because each department was focusing on practical concerns.

I certainly don't have a formula for preventing this kind of waste other than to suggest that: (1) HMOs are replete with potential research projects; (2) not a great deal of extra time is required to develop an experimental design and collect data; and (3) publishing is not too much of a problem, especially since at least three publications in the prepaid sector run mental health articles, not to mention the friendly editorial policy of many journals toward HMO-based articles.

If HMO mental health providers can appreciate the advantage they have in getting their work published, then they, rather than HMO management, may be the initiators of a system of improved communication in the field. Regardless of who initiates this system, management or providers, the end result will benefit all those involved in the prepaid sector.

NEED FOR HMO PRESENCE IN EDUCATION

From the point of view of one who evaluates applicants for prepaid mental health positions, I can see a problem: Most mental health professionals are not getting exposure to prepaid concepts and practice patterns in their professional programs. With few exceptions, the individuals I have interviewed for positions or evaluated during consultations have had little or no training in the modes of thought and work that will be essential in the new health care delivery system. Instead of being concentrated on populations and techniques of short-term therapy, the major focus of clinical teaching still seems to be on intrapsychic processes and long-term therapy. This simply won't do. Unless radical changes soon take place in the curriculums of professional programs, we will see a generation of professionally and personally dysfunctional mental health workers.

This educational lag also has serious implications for HMOs: They face the costly and time-consuming task of having to retrain almost all of their new mental health providers. To make matters worse, the prepaid sector's growth of 25 percent per year means that the problem is increasing at an accelerating rate throughout the field. If the prepaid sector's growth rate increases, which seems likely, then recruitment and training difficulties and costs will increase accordingly. The problems don't stop with recruitment and training, either; there are multiple secondary consequences of having to choose providers who are inadequately trained, including increased frequency of malpractice occurrences, low provider morale, and high provider turnover (see chapter 5).

Without doubt, major benefits would accrue to the field if appropriate changes in professional curriculums could be brought about. The time is now, but the question is how this should be done. There is reluctance, especially in psychiatric residencies and clinical psychology programs, to move from the status quo. Much of the resistance to change may spring from the fact that those who determine the nature of course material are often strongly oriented to private practice.

Obviously, there is no easy solution to this educational dilemma. Some HMOs have developed clinical clerkships, internships, and even residencies in one or two instances, but these programs are few, and they tend to have limited impact on the curriculum of the professional school itself. Our program usually has one or two students, who tend to work out quite well. However, I don't delude myself that our influence goes beyond the individual student; the training institution remains unchanged.

Perhaps the determining factor in bringing about the much-needed changes in the training of mental health professionals will be pressure from those who control the purse strings of psychiatric residencies and programs in clinical psychology, social work, and graduate nursing. If acceptable, efficient and cost-effective services are perceived to be lacking because of inappropriate provider training, then both state and federal legislators may find an incentive to act. If this happens, it would not be the first time that government policy influenced mental health service delivery toward a more "progressive" stance. During World War II, military psychiatry functioned by the dictum of return to function. Anyone who has seen film clips of therapy sessions or read case reports from this period cannot help being impressed by the quality and efficiency of service delivery then. Unfortunately, the techniques developed during that time never found their way into the mainstream of mental health training. In any event, a general reorganization of mental health training programs is long overdue in the United States, and it appears that the confluence of interest that is starting to develop in this area among providers, government, and the consumer may well bring about this change.

EXPLORATION OF THE CONCEPT OF PEER SELF-HELP

The ultimate goal of mental health work should be the elimination of the need for professional mental health workers. This ideal state is obviously far in the future, but there are signposts that can at least point us in the right direction. For example, focusing on the dysfunctional social unit, encouraging maximum self-reliance, and providing sociopsychological education to HMO members are techniques that foster autonomy and discourage dependency. These approaches are already being integrated into prepaid mental health service delivery with impressive results.

However, regardless of how elaborately or how extensively these techniques are developed, as long as the mental health professional is considered essential to their success, then the final step to complete autonomy for the emotionally distressed individual cannot be made. Some would say that this is not a "step" but rather a "leap of faith" for which there is little support. I disagree. Alcoholics Anonymous (AA), Emotions Anonymous, and Recovery, Inc., are only a few examples of peer self-help groups that have successfully made this leap. In effect, they have rejected professionalism, and their statistics are impressive.

Could the prepaid sector also make this leap? I think that it can, but the transition would most prudently be accomplished in increments or phases. Actually, most HMOs already have taken the first step in this process by referring menbers to AA. Some plans have gone further by having AA representatives conduct in-house meetings, and still other plans refer members to a wide variety of peer self-help organizations. The use of community resources by HMOs lends itself to the conceptual extension of peer self-help modes of treatment.

The next phase of evolving a peer self-help model within the HMO would be to develop therapy groups whose expressed goal is to become autonomous after a certain number of sessions. "Autonomous" must be qualified at present, because as long as the groups meet in the clinic, the department should provide at least periodic or "on-call" supervision. We developed two such groups over a one-year period that were quite successful. However, I must admit that my own anxiety level regarding their progress led me to intrude on their sessions more than once. The result was, of course, a mixed message to the group members: We have confidence in your ability to resolve your own difficulties, but . . . . Another element operating here was my concern about liability occurrences. Our attorney's opinion about this matter was not as clear-cut as I would have liked.

Potential medicolegal problems are probably the biggest stumbling blocks to developing a comprehensive in-house peer self-help program. If favorable rulings could be obtained in this area, then the prepaid sector would be free to explore this effective modality in detail. After all, the concept of peer self-help is entirely consistent with the core concepts of primary prevention. It is to be hoped that this issue will be resolved in the near future so that HMO departments of mental health can progress toward the ideal goal of mental health work.

DEVELOPING AN AIDS COUNSELING PROGRAM

It is impossible at this point in time to predict how extensive the AIDS epidemic will be in the United States. Some experts claim that AIDS will become, and will remain for many years, the central health problem of the world, and that it will bankrupt health care delivery systems around the globe. It has been estimated that the direct and indirect medical costs relating to AIDS will increase from a total of $949 million in 1985 to $10.8 billion in 1991.[19]

Whether these predictions are accurate or not, HMOs cannot afford to ignore the certainty that they will be called upon to treat large numbers of members who have contracted the virus. In other words, we should act as if there will be a large demand for our services and therefore prepare now to meet that demand.

Our initial move toward developing an AIDS counseling program should focus on our own knowledge of and feelings about the disease and those who have it. There is probably no other medical condition which engenders as much fear and hostility in the general public and in health care providers as AIDS. Therefore, acquisition of knowledge about the disease and resolution of our feelings about it are necessary before we can provide effective service to those who have been affected by the disease.

I have seen the effect on one mental health department that was called upon to treat an adolescent with AIDS. The response of staff fear predominated from the member's point of entry with the departmental secretary to the assigned therapist and even on to the inpatient unit to which the member was referred. Service to this member was fragmentary and less than ideal, to say the least. The overall tone of the treatment plan seemed to be, "Let's get this over as quickly as possible."

As a result of this experience, our deparmtent has scheduled a one-hour meeting every two weeks during which the entire staff reviews current AIDS literature, gains better control over feelings about the disease, and develops an AIDS counseling program within the department. In this manner, we not only learn about AIDS, but also anticipate and address the fears evoked by the disease. It has become clear to us in these meetings that a significant portion of our program will have to deal with the devastating effects the disease has on the family of the AIDS patient. Again, as in previously cited examples, concentrating on the "identified patient" will not be sufficient; the entire family must be considered when developing a treatment plan.

Viewed in its broadest context, much of this work will be in the nature of public health education. Although there are some who would disagree, I feel that public health education is a legitimate function of a mental health department if its goal is to deliver comprehensive service. After all, in the absence of a definitive treatment, education directed toward prevention is the only weapon against the further spread of AIDS.

Our next step along this line will be to bring other departments of the HMO into the planning process. A problem of such magnitude cannot be addressed effectively unless every sector of the HMO—clinical and administrative—takes an active part in developing the treatment program.

USE OF EMERGENCY DEPARTMENTS AS CRISIS/HOLDING UNITS

Even if an HMO doesn't own a hospital, it uses approved hospitals that have medical/surgical emergency departments (EDs). These departments have an untapped potential for acting as very short-term crisis or holding units. Most members who present to an ED in crisis and are ultimately hospitalized could be managed alternatively if some means were available to monitor and medicate them (if required) for a period of 12 to 24 hours. The ED is an ideal setting for this sort of rapid initial stabilization if a mutually acceptable agreement between the HMO and the hospital can be arranged.

The major problem in developing this kind of arrangement is the ED staff itself. Most ED personnel are not comfortable evaluating and treating emotionally disturbed individuals. They believe that so-called "psych patients" require an inordinate amount of their time and are unpredictable. The only way to allay the ED staff's apprehension is to provide in-service training in very basic techniques of evaluation, monitoring, and use of psychotropic medication.

Mental health in-service training of an entire ED staff is time consuming, but in the long run it is cost-effective. A well-functioning crisis/holding unit can reduce a plan's hospital bed days by 50 to 75 percent. Emergency department stays of 12 to 24 hours, followed by intensive follow-up on the ambulatory service or in a partial program, cost only a fraction of what the national HMO average length of stay runs. (For example, compare the cost of a 10-day hospitalization to the cost of 24 hours in a holding unit plus four or five crisis intervention follow-up visits.)

The community mental health sector has been aware of the advantages of holding units for some time. Community mental health center workers maintain that holding units not only cut costs but avoid most of the negative psychosocial consequences of hospitalization as well. I agree with this position. They do work and they do save money. This is only another example of a potential benefit to the prepaid sector that can come from careful observation of the community sector.

It should be noted that close liaison with the ED is necessary for these units to function properly. This linkage should start at the point the member enters the emergency system and continue throughout his or her stay in the ED. In other words, the HMO's mental health staff has to maintain communication with the ED staff regarding the member's progress and take an active part in discharge planning. It's no good simply to be told by phone, "Your member is ready for discharge—what do you want to do?" Face-to-face contact with the member should already have been made by departmental personnel and a post-discharge treatment plan developed. With this kind of liaison, the transition from the holding unit to the ambulatory or partial hospitalization service can occur with maximum efficiency and with minimum disruption of the member's life.

Appendix
SELF-EVALUATION

In keeping with the pragmatic, or "how to," tone that has been attempted in this book, the following two surveys will provide HMO managers or mental health directors with practical instruments by which they can evaluate the overall functioning of their departments of mental health. The surveys elicit information about the issues of greatest importance in the task of departmental evaluation—administrative structure, model of service delivery, staffing ratios and staff mix, provider productivity, and utilization rates, among others. These surveys were developed by the author and his associates in 1981 and 1982; they have been used successfully in HMO mental health consultation work from 1982 to the present. They also served as the basis for the most recent national HMO mental health survey, which has been referenced several times in this book.[2]

The first survey is designed for use with staff and group model HMOs and the second for IPA model HMOs. Questions are practical and procedural in nature and are self-explanatory.

In order to assess the mental health department's level of function, data supplied in response to the survey questions may be compared with survey data presented in the tables included in this book and with various recommendations made by the author throughout based on his experience. The tables are listed at the beginning of the book, and the author's recommendations on various subjects covered in the survey questions can be located by consulting the index.

Once it has been determined which operational areas require change, the survey can be readministered after corrective action has been taken as a means of evaluating how effective improvement efforts have been.

Staff/Group Model Survey of Mental Health Program

1. Name of HMO _____

2. (a) Age of HMO _____

   (b) Age of department of mental health _____

3. Model of HMO
   Staff _____ Group _____

4. Number of enrollees _____

5. Socioeconomic status of enrollees (show percentages)
   "Blue-collar" _____
   "White-collar" _____
   Medicaid _____
   Other _____

6. *Mental Health Staff*   *Full-Time Equivalent*

   (a) Psychiatrists   _____
   (b) Nonpsychiatric physicians   _____
   (c) Psychologists   _____
   (d) Social workers   _____
   (e) Psychiatric nurses   _____
   (f) Clerical   _____
   (g) Other (specify)   _____

7. Discipline of mental health director

   _____ Psychiatrist   _____ Psychiatric nurse
   _____ Nonpsychiatric physician   _____ Other (Specify)
   _____ Psychologist   _____
   _____ Social worker   _____ No mental
                                                health director

8. Are all members of the mental health department directly
   responsible to the mental health director? _____
   If not, explain _____
   _____

9. Does the mental health department have weekly staff
   meetings? _____ Other frequency (specify) _____

10. Staff clinical/administrative time in percentages:

                                  Percent   *Percent*
    Staff   *Clinical*   *Administrative*

    Psychiatrist   _____   _____
    Nonpsychiatric physician   _____   _____
    Psychologist   _____   _____
    Social worker   _____   _____
    Psychiatric nurse   _____   _____
    Other (specify)   _____   _____

11. Does the mental health department have quick, effective lines of communication with

_____ Providers in other departments of HMO
_____ HMO administration
_____ Attorneys
_____ Key community agencies such as protective services, emergency shelters, vocational rehabilitation, and Alcoholics Anonymous

Comments:

12. Does the mental health department provide in-service training for

_____ Mental health staff
_____ Nonmental health staff

Topics of in-service training:

13. Does the mental health department provide health education or health promotion classes such as parenting, stress management, weight reduction, and smoking? _____

Topics of classes:

14. Approximately what portion of the mental health department's caseload is referred by (show percentages)

_____ Self-referral
_____ Physician primary provider
_____ Nonphysician primary provider
_____ From outside the HMO (examples: employer, court, school)

15. Who triages patients for the first appointment (or reentry) in the mental health department?

_____ Assigned mental health therapist
_____ Mental health secretary
_____ Appointment clerk
_____ Other (specify) _____

16. What is the average waiting time for the following kinds of cases to be seen in the mental health department?

_____ Emergency
_____ Routine initial evaluation
_____ Follow-up visit

17. (a) Are any enrollees referred outside the HMO for mental health services? _____

(b) If referrals are made, under what circumstances are they made? (be specific)

(c) Who makes these referrals?
_____ Mental health staff only
_____ Mental health and nonmental health staff

(d) Are these referrals paid for by the HMO? _____

18. Approximately what percentage of mental health services are delivered by the nonmental health department HMO staff? (show percentages)

_____ Physician primary provider in HMO
_____ Nurse primary provider in HMO
_____ Other nonmental health department provider in HMO

19. (a) Are patients formally referred back to their primary provider for long-term follow-up after receiving mental health department services? _____

(b) Are these "back-referrals" made with the understanding that case management will be a joint (mental health and nonmental health provider) responsibility _____, or that total responsibility will be with the nonmental health provider? _____

(c) Are there specific criteria and procedures for these "back-referrals"? (explain)

20. (a) Is there a mutually agreed-upon therapeutic model used by the mental health staff in delivering services to enrollees? _____

(b) What model(s) are used?

_____ Traditional insight-oriented model
_____ Short-term, goal-oriented, problem-solving orientation
_____ Other orientation (specify) _____
Comment:

21. What is the total number of patient encounters in the mental health department in the past 12 months? _____

22. What percentage of the mental health caseload is seen in

_____ Individual therapy
_____ Group therapy
_____ Family therapy
_____ Couple therapy
_____ Medication checks
_____ Other

23. Group therapy data:

    (a) Type of groups (number of current groups in appropriate category)—

    Heterogeneous (mixed as to age, sex, problems, etc.) _____

    Homogeneous (special group for specific type of patient)

    _____ Couples group
    _____ Adolescent group
    _____ Children's group
    _____ Women's group
    _____ Divorced persons group
    _____ Substance abuse group
    _____ Other groups (list) _____

    (b) Number of time-limited groups _____
        Number of open-ended groups _____

    (c) Average number of patients in each group:

    (d) Are groups oriented toward the concept of peer self-help?
    _____

    (e) Does the mental health department refer to groups or agencies in the community that are free (or charge a nominal fee) and that promote peer self-help (examples: Alcoholics Anonymous, Emotions Anonymous, Recovery, Inc.)? _____

24. What is the average number of encounters per patient per year in the mental health department?

    _____ Average for individual therapy
    _____ Average for group therapy
    _____ Average for other types of therapy (specify) _____

25. Are psychometric tests used in the mental health department? _____

   (a) What tests are used?

   (b) Who administers and scores these tests? _____
   _____

   (c) Does the mental health department have criteria to determine need for testing? _____

26. (a) Approximately what percentage of patients receiving services in the mental health department are on psychotropic medication? _____

   (b) Who makes the determination as to whether or not psychotropic medication is indicated?

   _____ Psychiatrist
   _____ Internist
   _____ Nurse
   _____ Psychologist
   _____ Social worker
   _____ Other (specify) _____

   (c) Are regular follow-up appointments for medication checks made with a physician? _____
   Other staff? (specify) _____

27. (a) Does any member of the HMO mental health department have admitting privileges to an inpatient psychiatric unit? _____

   (b) What policies and procedures does the mental health department have for inpatient hospitalization in terms of (1) admission criteria, (2) screening of admissions, (3) arranging admissions, (4) monitoring patient progress and length of stay, and (5) discharge planning and discharge instructions to patient? (be specific)

(c) What is the average length of a psychiatric hospitalization for HMO members (days per episode)? ___

(d) What is the psychiatric hospitalization rate in number of hospitalizations per 1,000 members per year? _____

28. How is mental health service provided when the HMO facility is closed (nights, weekends, holidays)?

29. Does the HMO have any limitations of psychiatric inpatient coverage for the following categories of patients?

	Yes	No
Chronic alcoholics	___	___
Chronic drug abusers	___	___
Chronic mentally ill patients	___	___
Mentally retarded	___	___
Noncompliant patients	___	___
If so, please specify:		

30. Do you have special treatment programs for specific groups of patients (examples: partial program, residential program)? ___

Describe:

IPA Model Survey of Mental Health Program

1. Name of HMO _____

2. (a) Age of HMO _____

   (b) What is the contractual method by which mental health and substance abuse services are delivered? (examples: fee-for-service, community mental health clinic on a fee-for-service or capitation basis, private group on a capitation basis)
   Explain: (be as specific as possible)

   (c) If fee-for-service, what is the charge for:

   Individual therapy (full session)   _____
   Individual therapy (half session)   _____
   Family therapy   _____
   Group therapy   _____

   (d) If capitation, what is the capitation rate PMPM? _____

3. Number of enrollees _____

4. Socioeconomic status of enrollees (show percentages)
   "Blue-collar" _____
   "White-collar" _____
   Medicaid _____
   Other _____

5. Does the HMO have a designated person to provide liaison with mental health providers in matters of accessibility, membership satisfaction and complaints, appropriateness of psychiatric inpatient admissions and length of stay? _____

   If yes, what are the procedures by which this is carried out? (be as specific as possible)

6. Do mental health providers have quick, effective lines of communication with

    _____ Providers in other sections of HMO
    _____ HMO administration
    _____ Attorneys
    _____ Key community agencies such as protective services, emergency shelters, vocational rehabilitation, and Alcoholics Anonymous

    Comments:

7. Do mental health providers conduct health education or health promotion classes on such topics as parenting, stress management, weight reduction and stop-smoking for enrollees? _____

    If yes, give topics:

8. Approximately what percentage of the mental health caseload is referred by

    _____ Self-referral
    _____ Physician primary provider referral
    _____ Nonphysician provider referral
    _____ From outside the HMO (examples: employer, court, school)

9. Who triages patients for their first appointment (or reentry) with the mental health department?

    _____ Assigned mental health therapist
    _____ Mental health secretary
    _____ Appointment clerk
    _____ Other (specify) _____

10. What is the average waiting time for the following kinds of cases to be seen by a mental health provider?

　　_____ Emergency
　　_____ Routine initial evaluation
　　_____ Follow-up visit

11. Approximately what percentage of mental health services are delivered by nonmental health providers?

　　_____ Physician primary provider in HMO
　　_____ Nurse primary provider in HMO
　　_____ Other nonmental health provider in HMO

12. (a) Are patients formally referred back to their primary provider for follow-up after receiving mental health services? _____

　　(b) Are these "back-referrals" made with the understanding that case management will be a joint (mental health and nonmental health provider) responsibility _____, or that total responsibility will be with the nonmental health provider? _____

　　(c) Are there specific criteria and procedures for these "back-referrals"? (explain)

13. (a) Is there a mutually agreed-upon therapeutic model used by the mental health staff in delivering services to enrollees? _____

　　(b) What model(s) are used?

　　　　_____ Traditional insight-oriented model
　　　　_____ Short-term, goal-oriented model
　　　　_____ Other orientation (specify) _____
　　Comment:

14. What was the total number of ambulatory mental health encounters reported by all mental health providers in the past 12 months? _____

15. What percentage of the mental health caseload is seen in

_____ Individual therapy
_____ Group therapy
_____ Family therapy
_____ Couple therapy
_____ Medication checks
_____ Other

16. Group therapy data:

(a) Type of groups (number of current groups in appropriate category)—

Heterogeneous (mixed as to age, sex, problems, etc.) _____

Homogeneous (special group for specific type of patient)

_____ Couples group
_____ Adolescent group
_____ Children's group
_____ Women's group
_____ Divorced persons group
_____ Substance abuse group
_____ Other groups (list) _____
_____

(b) Number of time-limited groups _____
Number of open-ended groups _____

(c) Average number of patients in each group:

(d) Are groups oriented toward the concept of peer self-help?
_____

(e) Do the mental health providers refer to groups or agencies in the community that are free (or charge a nominal fee) and that promote peer self-help (examples: Alcoholics Anonymous, Emotions Anonymous, Recovery, Inc.)? _____

17. What is the average number of encounters per mental health patient per year in the following categories?

_____ Average for individual therapy
_____ Average for group therapy
_____ Average for other types of therapy (specify) _____

18. Are psychometric tests used by the mental health provider?

_____

(a) What tests are used?

(b) Who administers and scores these tests? _____
_____

(c) Do the mental health providers have criteria to determine need for testing? (specify)_____
_____
_____

19. (a) Approximately what percentage of patients receiving mental health services are on psychotropic medication? _____

(b) Who makes the determination as to whether or not psychotropic medication is indicated?

_____ Psychiatrist
_____ Internist
_____ Nurse
_____ Psychologist
_____ Social worker
_____ Other (specify) _____

(c) Are regular follow-up appointments for medication checks made with a physician? _____
Other (specify) _____

20. (a) Do the mental health providers who render ambulatory care also render inpatient psychiatric care if a member is hospitalized? _____

(b) What policies and procedures do the mental health providers have for inpatient hospitalization in terms of (1) admission criteria, (2) screening of admissions, (3) arranging admissions, (4) monitoring patient progress and length of stay, and (5) discharge planning and discharge instructions to patient? (be specific)

(c) What is the average length of a psychiatric hospitalization for HMO's members (days per episode)? _____

(d) What is the psychiatric hospitalization rate in number of hospitalizations per 1,000 members per year? _____

(e) What is the figure for psychiatric hospital bed days per 1,000 members per year? _____

21. How is mental health service provided on weekends, holidays, and at night?

22. Does the HMO have any limitations on psychiatric inpatient coverage for the following categories of patients?

	Yes	No
(a) Chronic alcoholics	___	___
(b) Chronic drug abusers	___	___
(c) Chronic mentally ill patients	___	___
(d) Mentally retarded	___	___
(e) Noncompliant patients	___	___

If so, please specify:

23. Do you have special treatment programs for specific groups of patients (examples: partial program, residential program)?

Describe:

References

1. Food for thought. *HMO Mental Health Newsletter* Oct 1985.

2. Practice characteristics and inpatient utilization: a national HMO mental health survey. *HMO Mental Health Newsletter* Dec 1986.

3. Mitchell SA. *Mental Health Services: The Case for Insurance Coverage.* Washington DC: Federation of American Health Systems (formerly Federation of American Hospitals), 1986.

4. Shapiro J, Sank LI, Shaffer CS, and Donovan DC. Cost effectiveness of individual vs. group cognitive behavior therapy for problems of depression and anxiety in an HMO population. *J Clin Psychol* 38:674–77, July 1982.

5. Berman M and McLaughlin M. Staffing patterns in the HMO mental health department. *HMO Mental Health Newsletter* Oct 1986.

6. Caplan RB. *Psychiatry and the Community in Nineteenth-Century America.* New York: Basic Books, 1969, p. 112.

7. Coleman JR and Kaminsky FC. *Ambulatory Care Systems,* vol. 4, *Designing Medical Services for Health Maintenance Organizations.* Lexington, MA: Lexington Books, D.C. Heath and Co. 1977, p. 267.

8. Patterson D, Bonstedt T, Green EL, Eichten JG, Bittker TE, Ryan H, and Pincus H. Report of the American Psychiatric Association's task force on health maintenance organizations, part I. *HMO Mental Health Newsletter* Mar 1986.

9. Patterson D. Psychiatric hospitalization of HMO patients. *HMO Mental Health Newsletter* Nov 1986.

10. Bittker T. Key concepts in prepaid mental health service delivery. *HMO Mental Health Newsletter* Jan 1987.

11. Mian P, Tracy K, and Tulcbin S. Expanded roles for mental health nurses within an HMO. *Hosp Community Psychiatry* 32: 727–729, Oct 1981.

12. Levin BL, Glasser JH, and Roberts RE. Changing patterns in mental health service coverage within health maintenance organizations. *Am J Public Health* 74:453–58, May 1984.

13. Rubin L. Design and operation of quality assurance programs. In: *Organizational Considerations in Developing Group Practice—Quality Assurance.* Washington DC: Group Health Association of America, 1977, p. 118.

14. Appelbaum PS. The expansion of liability for patients' violent acts. *Hosp Community Psychiatry* 35:13–14, Jan 1984.

15. Bonstedt T, and McSweeney JEJ. Interpretation of psychiatric exclusions in HMOs. *HMO Mental Health Newsletter* Sept 1985.

16. Califano JA. *America's Health Care Revolution.* New York: Random House, 1986, p. 19.

17. Galanter M. Self-help large-group therapy for alcoholism: a controlled study. *Alcoholism: Clin Exper Res* 8:16–23, Jan-Feb 1984.

18. Bonstedt T. When and where should we hospitalize alcoholics? *Hosp Community Psychiatry* 35:1038–40, Oct 1984.

19. Scitovsky AA, Rice DP. Estimates of the direct and indirect costs of acquired immunodeficiency syndrome in the United States, 1985, 1986 and 1991. *Public Health Rep* 102:5–17, Jan-Feb 1987.

INDEX

W